LEARN SOFT TISSUE MANIPULATION SKILLS

The Medical Massage Practitioner's Guide

Awilda Pelaez

LEARN SOFT TISSUE MANIPULATION SKILLS:
The Medical Massage Practitioner's Guide
www.AwildaPelaezLMT.com
Copyright © 2022 Awilda Pelaez

Paperback ISBN: 979-8-844130-10-6

All rights reserved. No portion of this book may be reproduced mechanically, electronically, or by any other means, including photocopying, without permission of the publisher or author except in the case of brief quotations embodied in critical articles and reviews. It is illegal to copy this book, post it to a website, or distribute it by any other means without permission from the publisher or author.

Medical Disclaimer
The book and website is not designed to, and does not, provide medical advice. All content, including text, graphics, images, and information available on or through this book and website are for general informational purposes only.

The content is not intent to be substitute for professional medical advice, diagnosis or treatment. Never disregard professional medical advice, or delay in seeking it, because of something you have read in this book or website. Never rely on information in this book or website in place of seeking professional medical advice.

The owner of this book and website is not responsible or liable for any advice, course of treatment, diagnosis or any other information, services or products that you obtain through this book or website. You are encouraged to consult with your doctor with regard to information contained on or through this book and website. You are encouraged to review the information carefully with your professional healthcare provider.

Publisher
10-10-10 Publishing
Markham, ON Canada

Printed in Canada and the United States of America

I dedicate this book to all healthcare workers, massage therapists, massage therapist students, and anyone who is open to learning and wants to improve and acquire new skills and techniques with curiosity, open-mindedness, and enthusiasm.

And of course, I dedicate this book to my dearest husband Cesar and my two amazing sons, Cristopher and Jonathan.

Table of Contents

Acknowledgments ix
Testimonials xi
Foreword xv

PHASE 1 1

Chapter 1: Establishing Your Practice 3
Scope of Practice 3
Ethics & Standards 4
Professional Boundaries 6
Approaches to Care 7
Hygiene & Sanitation 8
Positioning & Draping 8

Chapter 2: Set Your Treatment Time 11
Patient Intake Form 11
Client's Consent 13
Rates & Charges 14
Office's Policy 15

Chapter 3: Gather Information 17
Beside Manners 18
Indications & Contraindications 18
Massage Environment 21
Posture & Dysfunctions 21
Palpation 24

Chapter 4: Formulate Personalized Strategy and Not a Cookie Cutter 27
Who Are You Serving? 27
Keep in Mind Their Occupation/Job/Trade 29
Make an Assessment 29
Choose a Massage Therapy Modality & Technique 30
Customize & Individualize Treatment 32
Stick to the Treatment Plan But Be Flexible 33

Chapter 5: Body Mechanics 37
Type of Pain 38
Specialist Modalities 39
Compression & Friction 40
Trigger Point Therapy 41
Lymphatic Drainage Massage 41

Chapter 6: Target Areas 45
Targeted Massage (Address the Complaints) 45
It's More Than Just Anatomy 46
Separate Muscles From Everything Else 48
Breaking Negative Muscle Memories 50
Quality of Touch 52
Sequence and Flow 54

Chapter 7: Get Feedback 57
New Client & Standard Client 57
Importance of Comfort 59
Effectiveness & Benefits 60
Adjust Accordingly 61
How to Track Client Progress 141

PHASE 2 145

Chapter 8: Breaking the Patterns of Dystunction & Imbalance 147
Massage Routine or Evolving Treatment 147
Adaptation 148
Management of Complex Conditions 148
Analysis & Interpretations 150
Outcomes, Methods & Variations 150

Chapter 9: Listen, Observe & Feel 153
Subjective & Objective Symptoms 153
Measurement of Progress 153
Habits Contributing to the Current Situation 154
Treatment Plan or Referral Out 154
On Call or Not 155
Client Packages 155

Chapter 10: You Are Your Business 157
Results Get You Referrals 157

About the Author 165

Acknowledgments

I would first like to thank my husband, **Cesar Pelaez, for** supporting me during this process and encouraging me every step of the way; it's because of his love, patience, and support that I was able to get my book done so quickly. He is my best friend and the best husband. I learned so much from him and I am so blessed to be his wife.

I would like to thank my sons, **Cristopher and Jonathan Pelaez.** I would not have been able to achieve all my successes if not for their endless love, admiration, patience, and encouragement. Love you guys.

Thank you to my parents, **Santa Sanchez, and Maximo Capellan** and to my brother **Wildy Capellan**, my twin sister **Walkidia Gonzalez** and younger sister **Kenia Capellan** for their love and support. They are my biggest fans.

Thank you to **Kathy Palermo,** for supporting me and for treating me like her own daughter.

Thank you to **Leonardo Garcia**, for injecting faith into my heart and for being my spiritual father.

Testimonials

Awilda is an excellent medical massage therapist. I used to be disabled by lower back pain and I walked with a limp. Regular sessions with Awilda have changed all that, and now I walk upright, I can exercise regularly, and I am free from pain. Therapy sessions are cooperative and adapt to my current symptoms. But beyond that obvious stuff, Awilda teaches about how my muscle and tendon systems work, and why I end up in pain. She has shown me how to care for myself. Her professional attitude and serious attention to the whole patient is inspirational. I wish my doctor was this good.

Kirby M

I have been a client of Awilda Pelaez for the past ten years. This alone should be testimony to the positive impact Awilda has had on my health and well-being. She has a healing gift, using her skills and compassion to help others achieve wellness. She is a professional and extremely knowledgeable massage therapist, who consistently addresses presenting therapeutic needs, as well as providing a calm and relaxing experience. More importantly, I have found that therapeutic benefit has helped me with numerous medical challenges through the years.

Carmela J

For bonuses go to ...

Awilda is the best! I mean that literally; she has healing hands. I cannot thank her enough for giving me my life back. When I first went to Awilda in 2016, I was in so much pain and had limited mobility in my arm. My doctor, an Orthopedic Surgical Oncologist, wasn't sure I'd get full use of my arm after the bone tumor was removed. Awilda's positive energy and expertise about human anatomy helped to heal my muscles and made me feel better. Awilda's beautiful spirit, confidence and knowledge gave me hope that my arm would heal. As each week passed, my arm slowly gained strength and increased range of motion. My doctor is amazed by my progress. I truly believe that because of Awilda's help, my body healed, and I am pain free! I am so grateful for all she did to improve the quality of my life. Life without pain is a blessing. I am forever grateful for her. Awilda has a special gift for healing!

Kathy B

I first met Awilda through the recommendation of a friend. My friend is a semi-professional athlete and knows the importance of keeping a healthy body. The first time I met Awilda I was amazed at her knowledge of human anatomy and her passion to help people. At the start of our session Awilda asked questions to evaluate my problem. She then explained in detail what was going on with my body. Once her assessment of the troubled area was complete, she began to treat me as if she had x-ray glasses. At the end of each session, I felt like I could take on the world. Awilda is truly a gifted therapist who loves what she does. You can tell by her infectious personality. I will forever be grateful for meeting her because she changed my life for the better.

Marc C

It's my firm belief that we are all here for a reason. And I'm equally firm in my belief that Awilda Pelaez is here to be a living conduit for healing and hope. From the moment I met her four years ago for an injured back, I knew that I was in good hands. Literally. I've nicknamed her hands "heat-seeking missiles" that land, with precision, on the source of my tension and pain. It's my sincere hope that more therapists learn from Awilda because there are so many of us in need of her talents, techniques, and reassurance that it's once again possible to be pain free.

Elizabeth C

It's funny when people ask you how you're feeling, it's just a greeting. But when Awilda asks, you think more deeply about it, because her healing mind really needs and wants to know; it informs how she begins her treatment. I've been a grateful patient of Awilda's for many years after she helped me regain full range of motion in my shoulder and avoid cervical fusion surgery. I really look forward to going to a treatment, because while it will probably be painful and uncomfortable, I know it's freeing up uncooperative muscles that are throwing my body out of balance. With her gentle sense of humor, we always laugh through the painful parts together. The end always justifies the means.

Peter C

Foreword

Are you a medical massage therapist who is frustrated and discouraged, and possibly thinking about quitting the profession? Are you in search of more than simple answers to the complex challenges you face in this profession? Do you need understanding and a helping hand to guide you through the process of creating and establishing a profitable career?

Over her years in practice as a successful medical massage therapist, Awilda Pelaez has talked to dozens of therapists who have felt the same way. If you are looking to be inspired to grow your business to the next level, and be recognized and appreciated for your skills, *Learn Soft Tissue Manipulation Skills* is the book for you!

In this book you will find new skills and proven techniques to address your patients' complaints of pain and dysfunction, including:

- perfecting skills in bedside manners
- making accurate assessments
- formulating personalized treatment strategies
- getting referrals from your happy clients

Awilda has utilized these concepts, activities and processes in her private practice for more than 10 years.

For bonuses go to www.AwildaPelaezLMT.com

Being relevant, knowledgeable, skillful, and respected in this industry are the most essential components of a successful practice. I hope this book finds a prominent place in your treatment room for many years to come.

Raymond Aaron
***New York Times* Bestselling Author**

PHASE 1

Chapter 1

Establishing Your Practice

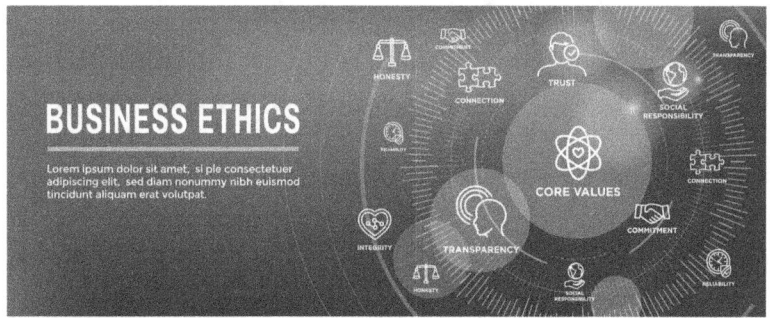

Scope of Practice

I am licensed in New York State, and in my state, massage therapists are licensed as health care professionals and have the same responsibility to provide assessment and treatment services within their scope of practice as do other health professionals, e.g., physicians, nurses, physical therapists. Practicing in NYS without a massage therapist license is a class E felony punishable by up to four years in prison, under the New York education law 7801 and 7802.

For bonuses go to ...

I urgently recommend you find what the scope of practice is in your state or country. And I encourage you to keep records of your updated license(s) and continue education courses just in case you get randomly audited.

Scope of practice refers to the things a healthcare professional is allowed to do under their license and is clearly defined by national standards in the United States to protect the health, safety, and welfare of the public.

Massage therapists will accurately inform clients, other health care practitioners and the public regarding the scope of their discipline and will represent their personal qualifications honestly, including education, experience, and professional affiliations upon request or in advertising.

Massage therapists may work in one or more of the following areas: therapeutic or relaxation massage: to promote wellbeing, improve sleep, treat anxiety, tension, and enhance a range of systemic body functions such as circulation.

Massage therapists also have a fiduciary responsibility to act on the best interests of their clients. Therefore, let us use our experience and knowledge to treat our clients honestly and confidently to the best of our abilities.

Ethics and Standards

Massage therapists must abide by professional conducts, principles, and guidelines. They are the behaviors, manners, and attitudes we must have every time with each client. The codes of ethics and standards of practice are as follows:

- Commitment to high quality of service
- Commitment to do no harm
- Commitment to honest representation of qualifications
- Commitment to uphold the inherent worth of all individuals
- Commitment to respect client dignity and basic right
- Commitment to informed consent
- Commitment to confidentiality
- Commitment to personal & professional boundaries
- Commitment to honesty in business
- Commitment to professionalism

Professional ethics is also defined as the principle that governs the behavior of the person or group business environment. Like values, professional ethics provide rules on how a person should act toward other people and institutions in such an environment. These principles are: principles of justice, principle of beneficiation, principles of nonmaleficence, principles of accountability, principle of fidelity, principle of autonomy, and principles of veracity.

In addition, your professional relationship with each client must be strictly confidential, respecting above all his/her rights to privacy. You must also adhere to the therapeutic treatment's boundaries, which include transfer counter, transfer dual relationship informed, consent right of refusal and scope of practice.

Additionally, the principles incorporating the characteristic and value that most people associate with ethical behavior are:

honesty, integrity, promised keeping, trustworthiness, loyalty, fairness, concern for others, respect for others, law abounding, commitment to excellence, leadership, reputation, morals, and accountability.

I hope you always strive to be a person of excellence and of great character, with outstanding behavior, good intentions, and fullness of integrity. Our clients rely on us and seek our services to get better. We should never abuse this trust and confidence!

Professional Boundaries

There is a very thin line between what's ethical and what's legal and you have to be careful not to cross it. As a massage practitioner it is crucial to keep boundaries. The most common boundaries are:

Physical Boundaries: you can create limits on how and when you are touched. As well as who you're comfortable touching.

Emotional or Mental Boundaries: protect your right to have your own feelings or thoughts, to not have your feelings criticized or invalidated, or not having to take care of other people's feelings.

Professional Boundaries: are the limits to the relationship of a member, or staff and a person in their care which allow for safe, therapeutic connection between the staff member and that patient, protecting both the staff and patient.

Social Boundaries: are objective forms of social differences manifested in unequal access to and unequal distribution of resources and social opportunities.

Time Boundaries: the beginning and ending of a block of time set aside for a particular activity.

Intellectual Boundaries: refer to thoughts and ideas. Includes respect for others' ideas and awareness of appropriate discussions. Intellectual boundaries are violated when someone belittles or dismisses another person's thoughts and ideas.

Boundaries are simply defined as the limit between acceptable and unacceptable behavior. Boundaries are rules and limits that help provide safety and protection to both the client and the therapist.

I highly recommend you to have a set of established professional boundaries for your practice when you are either on the phone, the treatment or communication with your patients.

Approaches to Care

Now that you are aware of the scope of practice, ethics & standards, and professional boundaries, and you follow these prerequisites, you are ready to assess and treat.

The main goal is having the client in a resting position and comfortable. Here are the basic steps: check the height of the table, check if the bed is warm, check if the room temperature is comfortable, and use pillows or a bolster for body support.

Hygiene and Sanitation

The hygiene and sanitation of your office space and treatment room(s) are essential and crucial to maintain a healthy environment, and prevent diseases, viruses, and germs. Make sure to change the sheets, table covering and pillowcases, and to clean and disinfect any surface that the client has touched to prepare for the next appointment.

As a massage therapist, you also need to maintain personal hygiene to minimize your risk of infection and also enhance your overall health. These are basic personal hygiene habits: Bathe regularly. Wash your body and your hair often, use deodorant, trim your nails, wash your hands, wear clean clothes, brush your teeth, use mouthwash.

Regardless of the dress code for your place of business, it is essential that your personal appearance matches the level of your professionalism. Clients do pay attention and so should we!

In addition, under the United State Department of Labor there is an Occupational Safety and Health Administration (OSHA). Its mission is to ensure safe and healthful working conditions for workers by setting and enforcing standards and by providing training, outreach, education, and assistance. Make sure to research and be informed of your local regulations in your state or country.

Positioning and Draping

First and foremost, draping is to protect the client's privacy. Throughout the massage he/she should feel covered, warm, and comfortable. After the client consultation, the massage therapist will leave the room so he/she can get undressed to his/her level of comfort. The client then gets between the fitted sheet and top sheet.

I recommend that you use sheets and blankets instead of a towel to cover the client because they are wider and offer more coverage and comfort. I believe the client feels more relaxed and less embarrassed to be undressed under the covers. A tensed body makes our job more difficult. So, our goal is to have our client nice and comfortable and relaxed.

To start your treatment, you can position the client depending on his/her needs, physical condition, or disability. You could start in a supine position (face up) or prone position (face down).

In addition, using your body properly in the administration of massage is essential. Proper body mechanics and posture is important for massage therapists because it helps in avoiding injury, fatigue, and helps make the best use of the massage therapist's energy.

For bonuses go to www.AwildaPelaezLMT.com

Notes

Chapter 2

Set Your Treatment Time

Patient Intake Form

The importance of an intake form is to collect information from your client to understand his/her condition, medical history, medications, allergies, and contraindications. I recommend that you use just a few key questions in your intake form so as not to overwhelm the client and also, I recommend that you be proactive by sending it ahead of time. You can use software that fits your needs, but please do not forget to have this form signed on file for your records and to keep their signature as a reading consent for treatment (s) so you can protect yourself if there is any future dispute.

Now with the completed intake form at hand you can prepare by reviewing the information before the appointment and have a better idea for their treatment, plus more time to focus on the first consultation. Also, remember to always review the intake form with them to make sure the listed information is correct. Keep in mind that there is always a chance of some non-mentioned issues and complications that can flourish during the first treatment. Some conditions may change for better or worse.

Massage therapists and other health care professionals often use SOAP notes to document clients' health records.

SOAP stands for a four-step note-taking process:

- **Subjective**: what the client tells you.
- **Objective**: observable data (posture, muscle tone, ROM, temperature, tenderness, swelling, etc.)
- **Assessment**: analyzing of client response to treatment and progress towards goals.
- **Plan**: includes your plan for their next visit and any instructions that you gave the client. Like recommendations for follow up visit (s). For example: treatments twice a week up to four times a week, stretching, and the use of heat or cold pads.

Make sure all SOAP notes, for every massage treatment, are signed and dated. Writing good notes, monitoring the progress, and keeping good records are vital in the clinical care process. By collecting all the necessary information, you will help improve with more accuracy the treatment plans of your client accordingly and based on their needs.

NOTE: this information is to determine the health impact of your treatment, not to diagnose your client.

Massage therapists will safeguard the confidentiality of all patient/client information, including patient/client records, unless disclosure is required by law or court order. Any situation which requires the revelation of confidential information should be clearly delineated in records of massage therapists. Be advised that the intake form can also be used for referral purposes. Keeping good records about the client's progress, their treatment goals, changes in their health, any adverse reactions, and response to treatment (s). Do not include your personal opinion. Only facts.

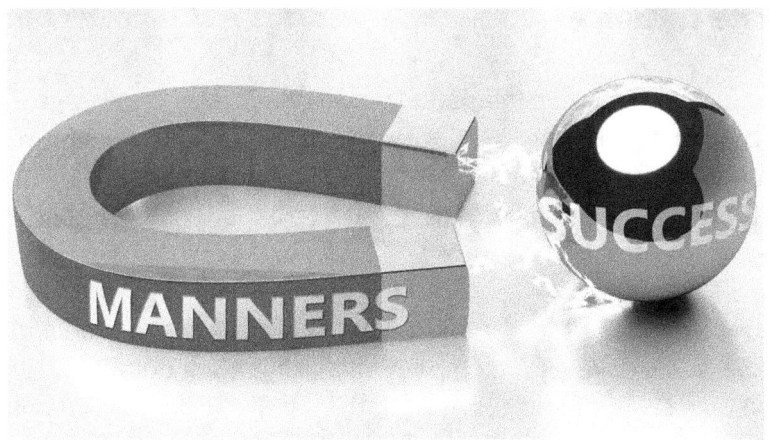

Client's Consent

Informed consent is a process by which a fully informed client consents to participate in the massage treatment. It originates from the ethical (and legal) right of the client to direct what happens to his/her body, and from the ethical duty of the therapist to involve the client in choices related to his/her wellness.

Having a signed consent in the file is a protection for the massage therapist. Think about your informed consent procedures and ensure that they are meeting the highest ethical standards by keeping clear communication between you and your clients.

For bonuses go to ...

In addition, massage therapists will respect the patient's/client's right to refuse, modify or terminate treatment, regardless of prior consent for such treatment.

Rate & Charges

In the United States the national average cost for a massage is from $85 to $150 per session, which could last between 60-90 minutes. The average national salary is from $43,000 to $115,000, depending on the therapist's experience and the type of massage.

Now, a massage therapist is serving only a client at a time and expects to make enough money to make a living doing massages. So, the biggest cost of the service is the human time that the therapist invests into that client. At the end of the day, you have to determine what is a profitable hourly rate for you and your business.

NOTE: only provide services you are qualified and licensed for.

In addition, to offering massage package deals is beneficial in terms of retaining customers and having a steady income. You can offer discounts to referrers and repeated clients.

I recommend that you establish your form of payment: cash, personal checks, credit cards, or health insurance. And when you do, make sure to have a good bookkeeping record and consult with your local Certified Personal Accountant (CPA) for more details.

Office's Policy

The following *policies* serve as a guide for our first-time and repeating clients:

- **For Record Keeping:** I use a daily signing sheet and progress notes (SOAP).
- **For Appointments:** I need 48 hours cancellation notice. Any lateness, less than 15 minutes will be deducted from the treatment time. Tardiness for more than 15 minutes will be rescheduled.
- **For Payments:** are due the same date of service.

It's understandable that in a case of an emergency some of these policies will not apply. But I keep very strict guidelines when it comes to my schedule and appointment time. "NO EXCEPTIONS!"

I find it helpful to hang signs in the office with my Office's Policies and to give courtesy calls to confirm a coming appointment or collect payments. I also use software that allows me to send email reminders and submit consents.

For bonuses go to www.AwildaPelaezLMT.com

Notes

Chapter 3

Gather Information

CLIENT INFORMATION: All information will be kept confidential

Awilda Pelaez, LMT
Medical Massage Therapy

Name_____ Date_____

Address: _____ City: _____ State: ____ Zip: _____

Home Phone: _____ Cell Phone: _____ Work Phone: _____

E-Mail: _____ Occupation: _____

Date of Birth: _____ Sex: M F Contact Lenses? Y N # massages in past? _____ How did you hear about us? _____

Why do you want a massage? _____

Have you ever been in an auto accident? Y N (Describe if yes): _____

List all the medications you currently take: _____

Who is your health care provider/MD? _____ Phone: _____

Describe any surgeries, broken bones, major injuries or accidents below--include dates (use back if necessary)
_____
_____
_____

Please check if you have had problems with any of the following:

- ☐ Sinus/Allergies
- ☐ Numbness/Tingling
- ☐ Sciatica
- ☐ Skin conditions/rash where _____
- ☐ Infections condition where _____
- ☐ Area of inflammation where _____
- ☐ Osteoporosis
- ☐ Seizures/Convulsions
- ☐ Dizziness/Fainting
- ☐ High/Low blood pressure
- ☐ Varicose veins
- ☐ Bruise easily
- ☐ Heart Condition
- ☐ Bursitis
- ☐ Arthritis
- ☐ Chest pain
- ☐ Shortness of breath
- ☐ Diabetes

NECK:
- ☐ Pain with movement
- ☐ Stiff Neck
- ☐ Grinding/Popping

HIPS, LEGS & FEET:
- ☐ Leg or foot cramps
- ☐ Feet feel cold
- ☐ Swollen ankles
- ☐ Ticklish feet
- ☐ Shooting pains
- ☐ Hip replacement
- ☐ Knee surgery

SHOULDERS:
- ☐ Can't raise arm
- ☐ Above shoulder
- ☐ Overhead

HEAD:
- ☐ TMJ
- ☐ Grind teeth
- ☐ Splint
- ☐ Headaches where _____
- ☐ Head feels heavy
- ☐ Loss of memory
- ☐ Lights bother eyes
- ☐ Ringing in ears
- ☐ Loss of balance
- ☐ Dizziness

ARMS & HANDS:
- ☐ Hands cold
- ☐ Loss of grip strength
- ☐ Shooting pains
- ☐ Shooting pains

LOW BACK:
Pain is worse when:
- ☐ Lifting
- ☐ Sitting
- ☐ Lying down
- ☐ Bending
- ☐ Coughing
- ☐ Working

ABDOMEN:
- ☐ Nausea
- ☐ Gas
- ☐ Constipation
- ☐ Diarrhea
- ☐ Tenderness

FEMALES:
- ☐ Pregnant
- ☐ # of weeks _____
- ☐ Menstrual pain
- ☐ Irregular cycle

Other conditions or information: _____
_____
_____
_____

(Please circle any areas of pain or injury)

PLEASE READ BEFORE SIGNING:

I understand that the massage I receive is provided for the basic purposes of relaxation and relief of muscular tension. If I experience any pain or discomfort during my sessions, I will immediately inform the practitioner so that the pressure and/or strokes may be adjusted to my level of comfort. I further understand that massage should not be construed as a substitute for medical examination, diagnosis or treatment and that I should be a physician, chiropractor or other qualified medical specialist for any ailment that I am aware of. I understand that massage practitioners are not qualified to perform spinal or skeletal adjustments, diagnose, prescribe or treat any physical or mental illness and that nothing said in the course of the sessions given should be construed as such. Because massage should not be performed under certain medical conditions, I affirm that I have listed all my known medical conditions and answered all questions honestly. I agree to keep my practitioners updated as to any changes in my medical profile and understand that there shall be no liability on the practitioner's part should I fail to do so. If I have a specific medical condition or specific symptoms, massage may be contraindicated and referral from my doctor may be required prior to service being provided. I understand that this clinic has a 24-hour cancellation policy and I will be liable for full payment for any appointments cancelled after this time. By signing below, I also authorize all employees and subcontractors of Awilda Pelaez, Suffolk County, to discuss and correspond about my medical status as it pertains to providing me with safe and effective massage therapy.

Client's Signature:_____ Date:_____

For bonuses go to ...

Bedside Manners

The ability to convey genuine concern about and interest in a client is an integral and inseparable part of the medical communications process. Good bedside manners can make or break a client interaction, either encouraging an honest discussion or putting off the client.

It may sound like a cliché but good bedside manners, being compassionate, empathetic, supportive, approachable, and friendly are not out of style, especially in a healthcare profession. A massage therapist's job demands good manners and professionalism at all times. The goal is to build a long-term business relationship!

Here are some of the actions to build a better bedside manner:

- introduce yourself and concentrate
- listen and ask open-ended questions
- make them feel comfortable
- use layman's terms as much as possible

Indications and Contraindications

There are 2 kinds of common contraindications that would prevent or restrict your clients from receiving a massage treatment: total, local or medical.

Total Contraindications: fever, contagious diseases, including any cold or flu, no matter how mild it may seem, being under the influence of drugs or alcohol-including prescription pain medication, Recent operations or acute injuries, Neuritis and skin diseases.

You cannot get a massage if you have these conditions because a massage could cause these conditions to flare up, making the problem worse. In addition, anytime you have a fever, whether from a cold, the flu, or some other infection, you should not get a massage. Massage increases circulation that may in turn help the infection increase the severity of the fever and the infection.

Massage can loosen blood clots. This could be dangerous because the clot could migrate to the brain, lungs, or heart. If you are aware of any blood clots, consult your doctor before a massage to make sure that it will not be affected by a massage treatment.

Local or Medical Contraindications: varicose veins, Undiagnosed lumps or bumps, Pregnancy, Bruising, Cuts, Abrasions, Sunburn, and Undiagnosed pain.
You should evaluate each client individually to identify and address any contraindications in accordance with their severity. Hopefully you can work around these areas. However, if they prove too severe, massage may not be appropriate. In that case, the therapist reserves the right to refuse treatment to ensure maintenance of health standards.

Please be advised that unless a massage therapist has been trained in prenatal massage, pregnant women should not have a massage treatment. It's especially risky in the first 3 months of pregnancy. If you are experiencing a health problem with either your kidney or liver, it is likely that massage will not be appropriate for you. Talk to a health care professional to see if massage will aggravate any kidney or liver condition. Massage can put increased strain on both the liver and kidney if they are not functioning normally. This occurs because massage increases blood flow, increasing the movement of waste through the body.

Cancer: Although massage is good at relieving some of the discomfort caused by cancer, it should only be given by someone trained to work with cancer patients. The patient should obtain a release form from his/her doctor to get treatment. If you have inflammation of any kind a massage to the area will further aggravate the situation. Uncontrolled Hypertension: Massage increases blood flow. If you have high blood pressure that is not under control, the increased blood flow that is a result of massage therapy may cause problems. As massage therapists we are exposed in detail to the benefits of a massage treatment; the key is to have some knowledge and discern when to use those techniques. Massage schools tried their best to give us all the tools to successfully achieve great practices. The indication of a massage treatment with the physical benefits of massage and myotherapy include: reduced muscle tension, improved circulation, stimulation of the lymphatic system, reduction of stress hormones, relaxation, increased joint mobility and flexibility, improved skin tone.

NOTE: follow protocols for any contagious disease and avoid putting yourself and others at risk.

The Massage Environment

Your office or treatment room needs to be cleaned and well organized. And to hold an immaculate environment of comfort, relaxation, and privacy. It is vital that your clients see and recognize you as a skillful and professional therapist. I recommend that, if possible, you display all your diplomas and certifications showcasing your education and achievements. This will help portray you as a relevant, educated, equipped and skillful massage therapist.

Every detail counts, from the quality of your sheets to the calm tone of paint and lighting in the room. Set the tone the minute the client walks through the door. Studies show that colors, lighting, and smells can actively relax. So, use these techniques to your advantage and do what you can in your practice to reflect your taste and personality. The point I'm trying to make is to make everyone feel welcome and peaceful from the beginning.

Posture and Dysfunctions

A great massage therapist **MUST** possess a keen trained eye to catch a poor posture or postural dysfunction, and sufficient training to know the source of the issue(s) and **WHERE** the body is compensating. Common posture problems are:

- **Forward head:** Forward head posture is when your head is positioned with your ears in front of the vertical midline of your body.

- **Kyphosis:** Kyphosis refers to an exaggerated curvature of your upper back (the thoracic spine) where the shoulders are rounded forward. ...
- **Swayback:** (hyperlordosis) and flatback (hypolordosis) and that's just it, it refers to the lordosis of your back! Your spine has natural curves, primary (kyphosis) and secondary (lordosis).

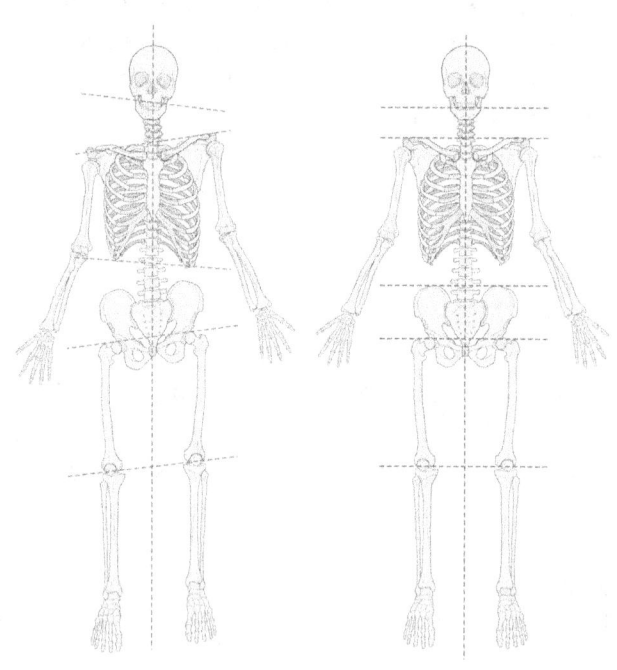

The skeletal system is **your body's central framework**. It consists of bones and connective tissue, including cartilage, tendons, and ligaments. It's also called the musculoskeletal system. In the skeletal system are gravity points to keep the body erect and balance in the correct position. Together with the Quadrants (a Quadrant is a quarter of an area, which in an anatomic structure may be divided by vertical and horizontal partitioning through its midpoint) they support your body's weight, maintain your posture, and help you move. There are four abdominal quadrants: The Right Upper Quadrant, or RUQ. The Right Lower Quadrant, or RLQ. The Left Upper Quadrant, or LUQ. and the Left Lower Quadrant, or the LLQ.

By looking at your client's posture and the way they stand you can find clues to determine which muscle (s) they are using to compensate for their dysfunction. In most cases these Quadrants and movement segments are part of the issue (s): ALTAS AND AXIS, C6 AND C7 VERTEBRAE, T12 VERTEBRA (THORACOLUMBAR JUNCTION), S1 VERTEBRA (SACRAL LUMBAR JUNCTION), KNEE AND ANKLES. The major postural and phasic muscles are the ones that compensate for any dysfunctions. Postural muscles act predominantly to sustain your posture in the gravity field. These muscles contain mostly slow-twitch muscle fibers and have a greater capacity for sustained work. They are prone to hyperactivity. Phasic muscles contain mostly fast-twitch muscle fibers and are therefore more suited to movement.

The main posture muscles are: Gastrocnemius, Soleus, Adductors, Medial Hamstrings, Psoas, Abdominals, Rectus Femoris, Tensor Fasciae late, Piriformis, Quadratus Lumborum (QL), Erector Spinae Group, Pectorals, Latissimus Dorsi and

Neck Extensor, Trapezius, Scalene, Sternocleidomastoid (SCM) Levator Scapulae.

The Main Phasic Muscles (Movers) are: Neck Flexors, Deltoid, Biceps, Triceps, Brachioradialis, Quadriceps, Hamstrings, Gluteus Maximus, Anterior Tibialis.

To gain an understanding of the postural balance, first locate which muscle(s) is involved in the postural dysfunction by palpating. Also locate the hyper mobility or hypo mobility because they change the motor function and are accompanied by temporary or chronic joint, muscular, and nervous system disorders by creating active and passive movements of the body. Also use landmarks that help identify lack of symmetry.

Palpation

The medical definition of palpation, (Latin word "palpare," meaning touch) is an examination by pressing with the fingers or hands on the surface of the body to feel the soft tissues or muscles underneath. As medical massage therapists our hands and fingers become our tools to evaluate the condition of those soft tissues and muscles. Let's not forget about the 4 Ts in the skill of palpation:

1. Tone
2. Texture
3. Temperature
4. Tenderness

Basically, what is being felt and what that might tell us about the acuity of the soft tissue and what to do about it. The goal is reaching a keenness of sensory perception with our hands and fingers, which is essential and one of the primary skills of our profession, our treatment and on-going assessment. You can develop and master this acuity by practicing until your touch helps you identify the soft tissue structures and conditions.

What we learn is to assess the somatic response of the body and identify other body parts such as ligaments, tendons, joint capsules, and muscles. The whole reason to get this skill is to improve your treatment and find the source of the pain so you can fix it.

For bonuses go to www.AwildaPelaezLMT.com

Notes

Chapter 4

Formulate Personalized Strategies and Not a Cookie Cutter

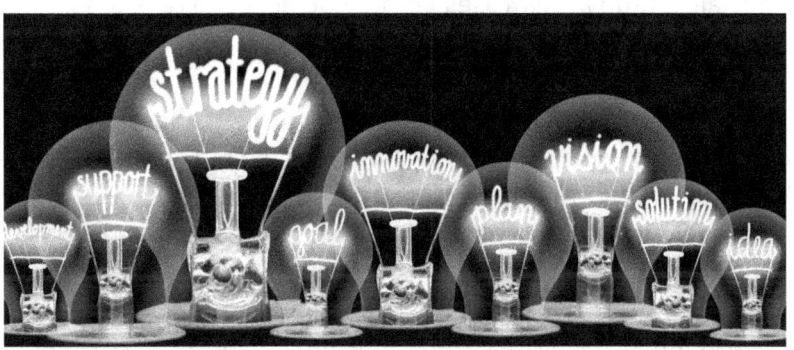

Who Are You Serving?
ex.: Senior, Athletes, Lifestyle)

Always keep in mind the following categories when you start treating a client:

1. age group and gender
2. illness
3. level of physical activity

4. health condition
5. sleep patterns and rest

Age is a huge factor. It may take a little longer than expected to see results because of other illnesses and medical conditions such as blood thinners, high blood pressure and diabetes but don't be discouraged you may be the answer to their problem. That's why they are there.

For clients with chronic illnesses, please get all their medical records and a referral from their primary care physician or specialist. Study their cases before you agree to do any treatment.

Athletes are one of the most challenging clients because they are short on time, always busy with no time to rest or keep them on track for their massage treatment schedule and, therefore, it is not possible to see desired results.

In most cases, clients who reach out for more therapeutic treatments have chronic conditions due to sport injuries and accidents. When they share their medical history, stay focused on the NOW current symptom (s) because you can be drifted away to an old injury and symptoms. For example: results of surgery and lack of physical activities.

Refer to in chapter 3 under *Indications and Contraindications about how to treat clients with medical conditions.

The importance of sleep is an important function that allows your body and mind to recharge, leaving you refreshed and alert when you wake up. Healthy sleep also helps the body remain healthy and stave off diseases. Without enough sleep the brain cannot function properly.

Keep in Mind Their Occupation/Job/Trade

Understanding the kind of job or daily activity your client does will help you identify the source of their strain(s), level of stress, pain and discomfort. It is important to know what they do every day and for how long they do it. For example: working in front of a computer, if their job is on their feet, or sitting for a long time. That alone will give you hints and clues of what's going on in their body or where their body compensates.

These are factors and clues. Pain and discomfort don't materialize for no reason. There is always an unknown reason: it could be a bad posture, a trauma related to an accident or a chronic condition. Usually, the biggest complaints of 90% of clients are: neck, shoulder, and back pain. All due to occupational hazard.

Make an Assessment

I recommend that you establish a protocol in how you make your assessment, so you can stay focused on the task. First, I will go over the intake form with the client, highlight any contraindications, and review medical records.

For every single visit always assess the client's range of motions (ROM), limitations, restrictions, and pain level (s).

Based on your findings you can now set a treatment plan. Determine the body position and what equipment you will be using. For example: cold and heat pads, Tens unit, or ultrasound.

After you determine the protocol and treatment plan based on where the body compensates and where you found the dysfunctions, make some suggestion how the treatment may go and connect with your client to trust you.

Use your judgment and communicate with your client what muscle(s) could be causing their pain. Share the treatment plan and the details with them. Use images, like an anatomy/skeletal poster. Also, mention the pressure you will be applying in different degrees so they can expect discomfort at times. The goal is to be able to mimic their pain because the battle here is pain versus pain.

Choose a Massage Therapy Modality and Technique

After you complete the client's assessment you are now needed to choose which technique or a combination of multiple modalities to use that will address the client's condition and provide them with the best results. Here are some massage modalities:

- **Swedish massage:** a gentle full-body massage. In summary, the 5 types of Swedish techniques are effleurage, petrissage, tapotement, friction, and vibration, which all encourage circulation and the softening of connective tissue.

- **Stress Relief massage:** activates the body on an internal level by decreasing the level of stress hormone and increasing immune cells. Swedish massage also relaxes muscles and increases circulation which all together results in a reduction of stress-related pains.
- **Hot stone massage:** relieves muscle spasm, pain, tension & improves muscle relaxation.
- **Aromatherapy massage:** used for a variety of different reasons, including relaxation, pain management, and improved mood. These are also some of the basic benefits of massage therapy. Adding essential oils is thought to enhance such benefits.
- **Deep tissue massage:** centers on realigning the deeper layers of connective and muscle tissue. It aims to release the chronic patterns of tension in the body through slow strokes and deep finger pressure on the tense areas, either following or going across the fibers of the muscles, tendons, and fascia.
- **Sports massage:** a form of massage involving the manipulation of soft tissue to benefit a person engaged in regular physical activity. The benefits of Sports Massage are widespread and can include: Increased muscle blood flow, raised muscle temperature, increased lymph flow and the removal of toxins from the muscles, breakdown of adhesions and scar tissue which builds up over time causing tension, and relieves muscular pain.
- **Reflexology:** a type of therapy that uses gentle pressure on specific points along your feet (and possibly on your hands or ears as well) to help you feel better. The theory is that this eases stress, and that helps your body work better. It's also known as zone therapy.

In addition, there is another technique called Shiatsu massage. This massage consists of applying finger pressure on various acupressure points in order to stimulate them and balance the body's energies (Qi). It is a holistic healing method, which helps balance the body's energy flows and consequently the process of self-healing. Shiatsu massages originated in Japan and relied solely on the use of finger pressure to certain points on the body, rocking movements, stretches, and joint rotations to re-energize the body. This form of massage is about the body as a whole instead of just focusing on one area.

Customize and Individualize the Treatment

I find it very import to customize and individualize massage treatment plans because it allows the client to recover in a way that is the best fit for him/her. Make sure to document the massage treatment plan(s), to identify and organize the medical issue(s) you want to work on in the massage treatment(s), what your goals for these medical issues are, and the steps you can take to work towards accomplishing good results and progress. Personally, this is the most exciting part of the whole process to me. Here you have the opportunity to shine and showcase your knowledge and skills. Do not be afraid to **BE ORIGINAL** with your methods and styles.

In addition, share your customized massage treatment plan and goals with your clients. Communicate your approaches and strategies with them and get them involved in their care.

Unfortunately, I hate to say this BUT there are some massage therapists that do not customize their massage treatments, but always use the same modality, the same routine, and the same technique in every client and every time. They completely disregard, ignore and neglect the client's needs and this is not acceptable!

I wrote this book with the intention to inspire you to strive and become the best massage therapist you can be. Not average, undisciplined, or careless. So, keep growing as a professional and reach all your goals in your business and career.

Stick to the Treatment Plan But Be Flexible

Remember, the treatment plan is the road map that a client will follow on his/her journey throughout treatment(s). On a journey, there is a chance of bumps in the road. The same is with the medical conditions of our clients. One day they could be feeling well in one area and worse in another and vice versa. Many factors can contribute to the slow progress or the appearances of new symptoms. Make modifications on the modalities and techniques that best serve the client at that moment. Do not be afraid to make changes. Focus your attention into finding a faster way to relieve their pain and discomfort. Now, be realistic and remember it took them years to develop this kind of complaints and chronic illness or the stress level. One visit might not be enough to correct it. Within the treatment plan, the massage therapist and the client will work together to determine the reasons for the massage. An honest conversation with your client is the key, and the goal is always the well-being of the client.

For bonuses go to ...

I will give you some scenarios and examples in the future chapters with graphics that can help you do the treatment more efficiently. The human body has multiple layers of muscles and is like pieces on a puzzle that we must figure out in order to restore homeostasis (balance).

Notes

Chapter 5

Body Mechanics

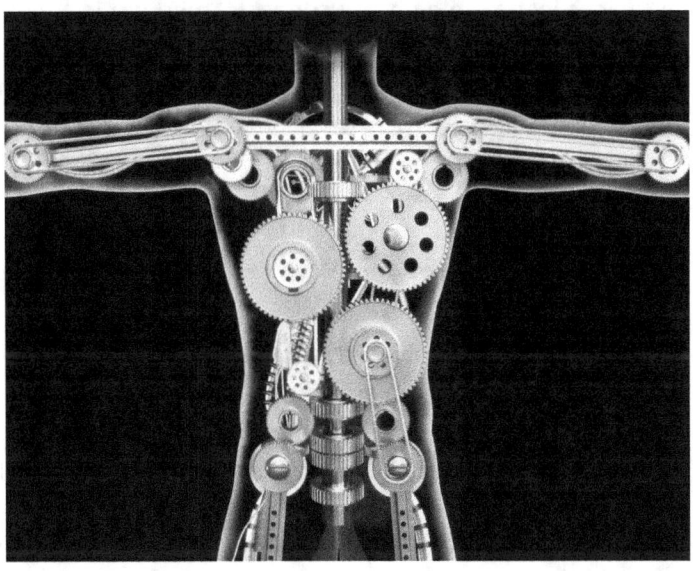

Body mechanics is a term used to describe the ways we move as we go about our daily lives. It includes how we hold our bodies when we sit, stand, lift, carry, bend, and sleep. Poor body mechanics are often the cause of dysfunction and pain in the body.

The minute a client enters your office you should check their gait. Gait is a person's pattern of walking. Walking involves balance and coordination of muscles so that the body is propelled forward in a rhythm, called the stride. There are numerous possibilities that may cause an abnormal gait.

There are 8 pathological gaits that can be attributed to neurological conditions:

Hemiplegic, spastic diplegic, neuropathic, myopathic, parkinsonian, choreiform, ataxic (cerebellar), sensory.
Look for clues and how the client is moving or compensating for their dysfunction, as every detail will help to determine what will happen during treatment. Here are some suggestions:

What is the type of pain?

- **Nociceptive pain:** typically the result of a tissue injury
- **Neuropathic pain:** pain caused by nerve irritation.
- **Acute (inflammation) pain**: an abnormal inflammation caused by an inappropriate response by the body immune system
- **Functional Pain:** pain without obvious origin but can cause pain

Describe the pain: Burning, sharp, aching, dull, stabbing, radiating, throbbing, and cramping.

Most of the clients have no idea of the body mechanic's dynamics, or our thought process as massage therapists in regard to choosing the best treatments for their condition.

I highly recommend that you learn, practice and be comfortable using the following **specialist modalities,** which require additional certifications:

- **Craniosacral Therapy** (CST): a gentle hands-on technique that uses a light touch to examine membranes and movement of the fluids in and around the central nervous system. Relieving tension in the central nervous system promotes a feeling of well-being by eliminating pain and boosting health and immunity.
- **Cupping Therapy:** an ancient form of alternative medicine in which a therapist puts special cups on your skin for a few minutes to create suction. People get it for many purposes, including to help with pain, inflammation, blood flow, relaxation, and well-being, and as a type of deep-tissue massage
- **Massage Chair:** an option to treat clients with disabilities. The chair massage is limited to the upper body; however, the benefits are similar to full-body table versions and include stress reduction, enhanced circulation, increased physical flexibility, a more vibrant immune system, pain relief, deeper sleep, and brighter mood.
- **Neuromuscular Therapy:** a modality whose goal is to recover from acute and chronic pain syndromes by utilizing specific massage therapy, like trigger point technique.
- **Manual Therapy/Sport Massage:** very similar to deep tissue massage because by applying deep pressure and targeting the muscles' deep connective tissues.
- **Myofascial Release:** a hands on gentle stretching (use in the right direction) to evaluate and treat the fascial connective tissue system.

- **Acupressure:** a traditional Chinese medicine art of balancing Chi energy.
- **Orthopedic Massage:** focuses on the treatment and prevention of musculoskeletal dysfunction and pain.
- **Petrissage:** applied using pressure to target the underlying deeper structures and to compress the muscles. Petrissage is more of an umbrella term as it consists of a number of movements and not just one such as kneading, skin rolling, wringing, picking up and squeezing.
- **Shiatsu:** a rhythmic pressure massage on a specific point along the body meridian using your fingers and elbows in a 3 to 10 seconds duration.
- **Lymphatic Drainage Massage:** gently assists the lymphatic system in maintaining the body's fluid balance.

Compression & Friction

Compression is a force that squeezes something together. Compression technique works best in bigger areas in the body and will produce results in areas like the anterior and posterior leg muscles (Quadriceps and Hamstring).

Friction is a massage technique used to increase circulation and release areas that are tight; particularly around joints and where there are adhesions within the muscles or tendons. Friction is defined as "an accurately delivered penetrating pressure applied through fingertips." **There are four types of friction:** Static friction, sliding friction, rolling friction fluid friction.

NOTE: Most of the benefits of these techniques are in a tendinous area, like the anterior knee.

Trigger Point Therapy

Trigger point in the skeletal muscles is a hyper-irritable knot, which feels like a taut band when compressed and produces referral pain. Trigger points are overly sensitive areas of tight muscle fibers and can be formed in the skeletal muscles after an injury, muscle overuse and even by psychological stress. When trigger points pain persists or worsens, some doctors call it myofascial pain syndrome. Keep this information in mind while working on a client who complains of pain for more than 10 days. Trigger point therapy can be used in the face, neck, shoulders, arms, hands, abdomen muscles, anterior legs, and posterior legs. Trigger points are confined in every part of the muscles in the human body. That's why I recommend that you learn the skill and technique of trigger point therapy in your massage treatment. I personally use this massage modality in my practice, and I can testify to the benefits and results of trigger point therapy.

Lymphatic Drainage Massage

The lymphatic system is a network of low-pressure vessels which provide a route for the return of interstitial fluid to the blood vascular network. A network of lymph ducts is present throughout the body. It moves fluids back to the circulatory system, while also providing important immune functions.

For bonuses go to ...

Lymphatic drainage massage will help with allergies, bloating brain fog, chronic lethargy, constipation, depression, digested problems, and swollen lymph nodes. Also, the circulatory system and the endocrine system encourage hormones to be secreted at the right time and in the right dose helping their functions.

Understanding body mechanics is the essential and vital skill that will help you excel as a successful massage practitioner. You may wonder why I am making such a bold statement but having been an experienced medical massage practitioner for over twelve years, I believe that my successful practice is a result of my sensitivity and common sense when I treat my clients.

Notes

Chapter 6

Target Areas

Targeted Massage (Address the Complaints)

Targeted massage is an approach to massage therapy that allows a massage therapist to address specific trouble areas of the body. Based upon the client's needs, the massage therapist will determine the best methods to relieve the pain and improve overall health.

Go over the intake form and ask the client where the pain is, and what their complaints are. Then you will assess their gait and range of motion (ROM), which will help you determine the plan of action for the massage treatment. Keep in mind which antagonist muscle is part of the problem. In an antagonistic muscle pair, as one muscle contracts the other muscle relaxes or lengthens. The muscle that is contracting is called the agonist and the muscle that is relaxing, or lengthening is called the antagonist. The agonist in a movement is the muscle(s) that provides the major force to complete the movement. Because of this, agonists are known as the 'prime movers.' For example: In the bicep curl which produces flexion at the elbow, the biceps muscle is the agonist.

I recommend that you prepare the trouble area(s) using heat to increase the circulation or ice to calm the nerve and reduce pain. Then, palpate the trouble area (s) to make sure where the origin of the problem is. The key is finding the source of the problem and where it is related to the symptoms.

Please refer to the chapter on body mechanics for more information.

It's More Than Just Anatomy

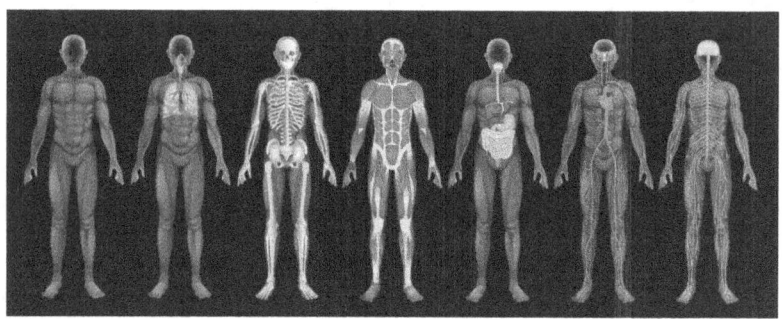

Anatomy and physiology are two of the most basic terms and areas of study in the life sciences. **Anatomy** refers to the internal and external structures of the body and their physical relationships, whereas **physiology** refers to the study of the functions of those structures.

The human body is made up of all the living and nonliving components that create the entire structure of the human organism, including every living cell, tissue, and organ. On the outside human anatomy consists of the five basic parts: head, neck, torso, arms, and legs.

The human body is composed of many systems, like an orchestra working in harmony. One of the struggles most massage therapists have is grasping the depth and vastness of the multiple components of the human body. Here are some facts: there are 650 muscles in the human body, 360 joints in adults, 900 ligaments dense and collagen fibers, 206 bones (long and short) as an adult, 78 organs, billions of neurons, 33 vertebrae, and 6.5 liters of blood.

Massage therapists with knowledge of **kinesiology** can work any muscle group to aid relaxation, loosen contracted muscles, and soothe an overworked body. Kinesiology focuses on three muscle movements: In a **Concentric contraction**, the force generated by the muscle is less than the muscle's maximum, and the muscle begins to shorten. This type of contraction is widely known as muscle contraction. It requires more energy compared to the other two types, but this contraction generates the least force. **Isometric exercises** are tightening (contractions) of a specific muscle or group of muscles. During isometric exercises, the muscle doesn't noticeably change length. The affected joint also doesn't move. Isometric exercises help maintain strength. They can also build strength, but not effectively. An **Eccentric** (lengthening) muscle contraction occurs when a force applied to the muscle exceeds the momentary force produced by the muscle itself, resulting in the forced lengthening of the muscle-tendon system while contracting.

For bonuses go to ...

In addition, a massage therapist needs to understand the following **aspects of anatomy** in order to effectively help their clients: Body plan, fascia, joints, kinesiology, lymph system, medical terms, wellness terms, muscles and muscles' actions and the systems of the human body.

Massage therapists must have a comprehensive understanding of anatomy. Not only is it important to know the muscular system — muscle attachments and actions — and skeletal system, but it is also important to understand how massage affects the body systemically. When massage therapists have a full understanding of the functions of the body, they are able to provide their clients with the most beneficial and safe massage.

Separate Muscles From Everything Else

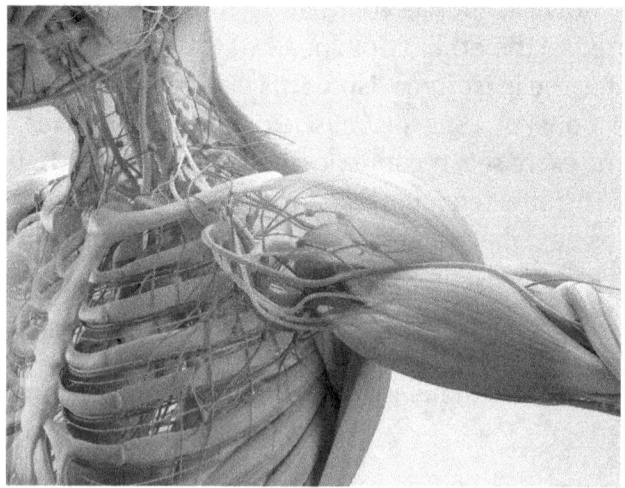

Each muscle is surrounded by a connective tissue sheath called the epimysium. Fascia, connective tissue outside the epimysium, surrounds and separates the muscles. Massage therapy relaxes muscle tissue, which reduces painful contractions and spasms. Massage can also reduce nerve compression. To understand this, consider that when muscles are contracted, they sometimes compress the nerves around them.

The most common causes of muscle pain are tension, stress, overuse, and minor injuries. This type of pain is usually localized, affecting just a few muscles or a small part of your body. Massage helps relieve tightness in the muscles by increasing blood circulation to the muscles. Restoring circulation to the muscles increases new blood cells to the area, stimulating the healing process. Massage relaxes the muscles, separating and loosening muscle fibers and speeding up the delivery of the nutrients they need to function properly while disposing of metabolic waste that can cause pain and delay recovery. **Lactic and uric acid** build up around muscles, causing pain, soreness, and lack of flexibility.

Massage releases these compounds in the bloodstream and when they are excreted from the body, lowering its overall acidity. Massage also releases creatine, which is a natural byproduct of muscle use and strain. Massaging knotted muscles helps to release that buildup and increase blood flow, providing oxygen to parts of the muscle that weren't getting enough before.

When a muscle is in pain the body protects itself by avoiding that area and compensating with another area. This is how dysfunctions are created, and it's our job to work in these areas of pain and discomfort. Be gentle in your application and approach plus communicate your intentions while working with your clients. Tell them why you are doing what you are doing!

Breaking Negative Muscle Memories

Muscle memory is a neurological process that allows you to remember certain motor skills and perform them without conscious effort. Skill retention from muscle memory can potentially last forever, barring any neurological or physical ailments.

Muscle memory is also the act of committing a specific motor task into memory through repetition. While your muscles themselves can't actually remember anything, they are full of neurons attached to your nervous system that play a role in motor learning.

However, since your muscle cells retain the nuclei they gained from previous training, you can typically regain these losses in little time. Bottom line: Your muscles do remember how big and strong they used to be—and they respond very well to training after time off.

In addition, the dictionary definition of muscle memory is the ability to reproduce a particular movement without conscious thought, acquired because of frequent repetition of that movement. The term itself is a misnomer because when a muscle is not connected to the brain it cannot perform, and the opposite is correct too. **Muscle memory** of the **brain** — **Muscle memory** of the **brain** is actually the **brain** learning a motor skill. Thus, it should be called "**brain** motor" when the muscle is doing an action is the actual brain working. Muscle memory is just habits we have impregnated in our subconscious from when we were younger, and some of those habits can become second nature. Obviously, some of those muscle memories when they are bad habits can affect us physically and emotionally. Most of the time when a client or patient complains of aches and pain it is the result of bad posture, a wrong jerky fast movement, a trauma, or an injury.

It has been my experience that in most clients the pain will come gradually, and, in some cases, the pain will be a spontaneous episode, like a twitch. We cannot limit habits as wrong, good, bad, healthy, or unhealthy. But it is definitely good to also challenge the body to be more flexible and to build strength.

We also must keep in mind that the lifestyle of every client is a key to understanding the reason(s) for their pain. It is obvious that people who are very active are going to have more aches and pains than people with a sedentary lifestyle. When a movement is repeated over time, the brain creates a long-term muscle memory for that task, eventually allowing it to be performed with little to no conscious effort. This process decreases the need for attention and creates maximum efficiency within the motor and memory systems.

Muscle memory is a type of procedural memory, which is a type of implicit memory (unconscious, long-term memory) which aids the performance of particular types of tasks without conscious awareness of these previous experiences. Procedural memory guides the processes we perform, and most frequently resides below the level of conscious awareness. When needed, procedural memories are automatically retrieved and utilized for execution of the integrated procedures involved in both cognitive and motor skills, from tying shoes, to reading, to flying an airplane. Procedural memories are accessed and used without the need for conscious control or attention.

Procedural memory is created through procedural learning or repeating a complex activity over and over again until all of the relevant neural systems work together to automatically produce the activity. Implicit procedural learning is essential for the development of any motor skill or cognitive activity.

As medical massage therapists, we have to be familiar with how regular activities change the function of the muscles deep from a cellular level. The negative muscle memories need to be unlearned, untrained and removed from our clients' routines in order to bring healthy habits and progress.

Quality of Touch

A great quality of touch can only be achieved with empathy, intuition, and a genuine passion to help others feel wonderful. Many massage therapists fail to reach a great quality of touch because they believe they know the client's body better than they do.

Touch is very important because it stimulates the release of endorphins which help to decrease pain and increase pleasure and mobility. Massage increases blood circulation and relaxes muscles, allowing for greater range of movement in certain areas.

In addition, the quality of the touch most of the time will depend on the client's liking. Some people are very sensitive to deep pressure. Keep this in mind when you're treating a client and remember to ask their pain tolerance to avoid hurting them during treatment. Remember, it is all about the comfort of your client.

The first thing that every massage therapist student must master is the basic massage strokes. The four basic massage strokes are effleurage, petrissage, tapotement, and friction.

- **Effleurage:** (light or deep stroking) Gliding strokes with the palms, thumbs and/or fingertips.
* **Petrissage:** (kneading) is an effective massage technique in which deep pressure is applied to tissue and underlying muscle. Petrissage is used to free up movement of tissues and muscle by treating muscle knots or spasms. The petrissage massage technique uses a squeezing technique which can alleviate muscle spasm.
- **Tapotement:** (gentle slapping) is a specific technique used in Swedish massage. It is a rhythmic percussion, most frequently administered with the edge of the hand, a cupped hand, or the tips of the fingers.
- **Friction:** is a massage technique used to increase circulation and release areas that are tight; particularly around joints and where there are adhesions within the

muscles or tendons. Friction is defined as "an accurately delivered penetrating pressure applied through fingertips."

In a massage treatment clients can lie in several positions. When in the **prone position** a client is face down, in **supine** position a client is face up. **Side-lying** is also known as the lateral recumbent position. Side-lying position allows you to interact with these soft tissues and associated joints with more ease, accuracy, and stability. You will also be able to explore more unique and multidimensional movements when stretching and rocking spine, pelvic and pectoral girdle tissues.

The quality of your touch at the end of a session is important, too. End with a moment of focused touch and gently pull your hands from the body. This allows your client to continue to enjoy the effects of the massage without the jolt of an abrupt change of energy at the end.

Sequence and Flow

A sequence is simply a collection of individual techniques put together with the intention of achieving a specific effect or series of effects. Of the many massage sequences that are possible, the selection of techniques should, to a large extent, be determined by the specific treatment goals. Usually, clients need to change position at least once during a massage. It is important to sequence these changes based on client needs and wants, moving the client only to gain access to target areas during the session.

A flow is a sequence of steps that leads massage from one body part to another in a routine, continual pattern.
It can be a real challenge to keep a sequence and flow of movements while during treatment to effectively address the discomfort and to release pain. Based upon the client's needs, the massage therapist will determine the best methods to relieve the pain and improve the client's overall health.

For bonuses go to www.AwildaPelaezLMT.com

Notes

Chapter 7

Get Feedback

New Client and Standard (Regular) Client

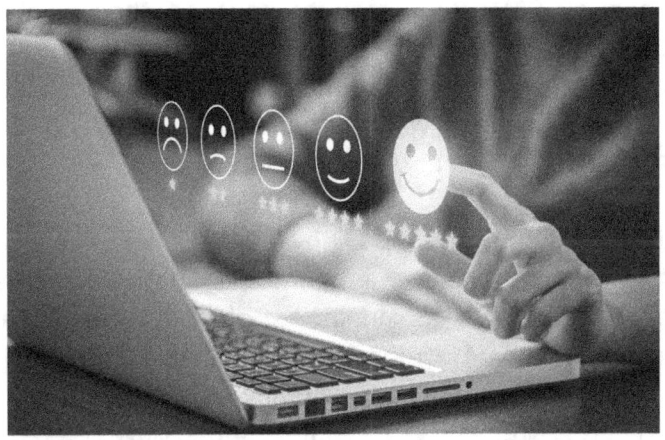

All clients start as a new client and those same new clients become the regular clients in your practice. The treatment of a new client represents an empty canvas, and the treatment of a regular client is the full picture.

As valuable as new clients are, your regular clients are actually the bread and butter of your business and income. Regular clients feel comfortable with you and trust you to continue to take care of them. They will continue treatment with you, even if it is just for maintenance.

An important part of being a good massage therapist is having **good communication skills**. Being articulate starts with active listening. You must listen as much as you speak. Make sure the client clearly understands what you are going to do, and how they will feel after a massage. Communication and feedback are always the key to building a good connection and trust. Make sure to address all the client's concerns and needs from the very beginning and make them feel included in their treatment plan. Most massage therapists ask their clients to provide feedback during the massage so that massage techniques can be adjusted to the client's specific preferences and needs. Your clients will thank you and your practice will reap the rewards of your diligence.

It is also very important to be knowledgeable and skillful. A massage therapist must remember to provide good service and a great job as well as running a profitable business. These services include time, atmosphere, cleanliness, and convenience. Listen to what clients say, as many clues lie hidden here. Listen and grow your business. Have set, reliable hours, but be flexible and willing to work when clients need you, not always when you want to.

The bottom line is that we need to have satisfied and happy clients that keep coming back to us for treatments and results!

Importance of Comfort

Our responsibility as massage therapists is to provide relief and comfort. Here are a few useful tips and tricks you can use to make your client's massage a fully enjoyable experience: have a face rest, delight the senses with heavenly aromas, include hot or cold therapy, provide support for the shoulders, back, legs and feet and use a wide massage table.

Ensure that your client takes off only as much clothing as he/she is comfortable removing. And if he/she doesn't want to remove their clothing, ask them to wear clothing that will be comfortable during the massage and will allow you to touch and move the areas of the body that need to be massaged.

Working with a client with a **chronic pain condition** requires that massage therapists take inventory of how their body is feeling and adjust as necessary. Trigger point massage and therapeutic massage may relieve pain. In most cases, after an injury, a therapist may recommend massage once or twice a week throughout the client's recovery. This is typically recommended but it also depends on how the body feels. If the client has a chronic health condition, it is preferable to have he/she see their primary care physician prior to getting a treatment.

The goal of a massage treatment is to keep the client in a comfort zone, unstressed, unwind, loosen, relaxed, and decompressed.

For bonuses go to ...

Effectiveness & Benefits

Massage may often be perceived as a safe therapeutic modality without any significant risks or side effects. Massage benefits can include: reducing stress and increasing relaxation; reducing pain and muscle soreness and tension; and improving circulation, energy, and alertness.

Massage therapy is a proven method to help **combat stress** and reduce its negative effects on the mind and body. It has been shown that even just 10 minutes of massage therapy can activate the body's natural happy hormones and leave you feeling more relaxed and less stressed.

A relaxation massage is a smooth, gentle treatment that relieves muscular tension, increases circulation, and **promotes a general sense of relaxation.**

Therapeutic massage may **relieve pain** by way of several mechanisms, including relaxing painful muscles, tendons, and joints; relieving stress and anxiety; and possibly helping to "close the pain gate" by stimulating competing nerve fibers and impeding pain messages to and from the brain.

Massage therapy **relaxes muscle tissue**, which reduces painful contractions and spasms. Massage can also reduce nerve compression. To understand this, consider that when muscles are contracted, they sometimes compress the nerves around them.

Massage relaxes muscles by **increasing temperature and blood circulation.** An increase of temperature is stimulated by friction against the skin. Increased circulation delivers more blood to the muscles, removing waste products and relieving tension. Massage facilitates circulation because the pressure created by the massage technique actually moves blood through the congested areas. The release of this same pressure causes new blood to flow in.

Massage therapists can really benefit from using energy work in addition to their massage techniques. Clients **release energy**, often continuously, throughout the massage. People store their emotions, memories, beliefs and thoughts in their energy system, and massage allows them to come up to be released.

Massage **interrupts stress-inducing patterns** and helps to restore your body to a balanced state, thereby alleviating the mental block of stress from your mind and allowing you to dedicate energy to thinking and completing important tasks.

Massage is generally considered part of integrative medicine. It's increasingly being offered along with standard treatment for a wide range of medical conditions and situations.

Adjust Accordingly

Massage therapists must be flexible about changing the treatment plans in order to find a better solution to improve the client's health and results. Here I'm giving you vital knowledge and wisdom. Information and skills that I personally apply in my private practice and have made me the successful professional I am today.

I would like to cover each region of the body in more detail. This information will help you develop a deeper understanding of the soft tissue and the muscle behavior when clients are in pain, have wrong alignments, and body compensation.

Now, I would like to describe the definitions, mechanics and interpretations of the source of the dysfunctions (for muscle tissues) of the body from the head to the toes. As well as, to offer you solutions, massage modalities and techniques to help you address these issues.

THE HEAD (Skull)

The head is an anatomical structure that houses the brain and is the home of the face and the five senses. The head contains sensory organs: two eyes, two ears, a nose and tongue inside of the mouth. Together, these organs function as a processing center for the body by relaying sensory information to the brain. The head is an organ of balance, and it is the entrance of the respiratory system and digestive system which are fundamental to the sustainability of our life (breathing and eating).

The head is also called the nervous system and is composed of a central nervous system (CNS), brain and spinal cord, and the peripheral nervous system (PNS), cranial nerves and spinal nerves. The CNS is located within the dorsal cavity, and the PNS extends through the ventral cavity

Let's explore the face and neck as the *primary part* of the scalp muscles and the forehead. The *face muscles* control the face expressions. The *jaw muscles* open and close the mandible and the *neck muscles* support and balance the head on the spinal column, plus allow its movement in all directions.

The skull (head) consists of twenty-two cranial bones and only the mandible is movable. The temporomandibular joint function (TMJ) is like a sliding hinge connecting the jawbone to the skull. Its dysfunction can lead to terrible pain and discomfort. Muscles responsible for TMJ, are primarily the Masseter muscle, Temporalis muscles, and Pterygoids muscle, which we will cover in detail later in this chapter.

Muscles responsible for head and face pain: *Frontalis muscles, Occipitalis & Suboccipital muscle group, Orbicularis oculi muscle, Temporalis muscle, Zygomaticus muscles, masseter muscle, pterygoid muscles, and Sternocleidomastoid Muscle (SCM also a neck muscle).*

* **Frontalis Muscles**: the action is to wrinkles the brow. When there are trigger points in the frontalis muscle it can also transfer pain to the forehead producing a headache. The origin of this muscle is the Cranial Aponeurosis, and its insertion is the skin above the eyebrows. The nerve is Facial Nerve.

* **Occipitalis Muscle**: the action is the wrinkling of the forehead assists the frontalis muscle. When there are trigger points in the Occipitalis muscle produces pain as headaches in the posterior lateral part of the head, plus pain behind the eye. Its origin is in the Superior Nuchal Line of the Occipital bone mastoid part of the temporal bone and the muscle insertion is the Galea Aponeurosis,

For bonuses go to ...

and its nerve is the Posterior Auricular nerve (Facial Nerve).

* **Suboccipital Muscles Group:** are Obliquus capitis superior, Obliquus capitis interior, rectus capitis posterior major and the rectus capitis posterior minor. This group of muscle are mainly known as Suboccipital muscles.

    The action of this muscle group is to provide extension, side bending and rotation between the occiput and the C1 and C2. When there are trigger points in the Suboccipital muscles group they can cause an intense headache that penetrates the skull, making it very difficult to localize. Their origin is the occipital bone, and their insertions are C1 and C2, vertebrae transverse and spinous processes. This muscle group nerve is a branch of the dorsal primary division of the Suboccipital Nerve.

* **Orbicularis Oculi Muscle:** its action is to close the eyelids, intentional blinking, strong closure of the eyelids and squinting. Its origin is in the medial palpebral ligament, frontal and maxillary bones and the tissue of the eyelid (superiorly and medially of the eye orbit). When there are trigger points in the Orbicularis oculi muscle produces pain in the superior eyelid and down to the side of the nose.

* **Temporalis Muscle:** The action of the temporalis muscle is to close the jaw. Acting individually, this muscle will deviate the mandible to the same side. Headaches are common on this muscle due to the trigger points. The origin is at the Temporal lines on the Parietal bone of the skull and the insertion of this muscle is at the Coronoid

process of the mandible and its nerve is the Mandibular nerve.

NOTE: you should be examining and treating all clients complaining of headaches and TMJ problems. Palpate between the sphenoid bone and the posterior aspect of the temporal bone down to the zygomatic arch. Be advised that the temporalis muscle architecture is convergent, meaning their fiber direction varies from diagonal to superior/inferior. Other muscles to examine are the Masseter, Pterygoids, all facial muscles, and all anterior, lateral, and posterior neck muscles.

Manual Therapy suggestions: the client lies supine, stripping strokes downward covering the entire muscle, stroking across, looking for trigger points in temporalis muscle and pressing firmly until release.

* **Zygomaticus Major and Minor Muscles**: their action is to pull the corners of the mouth up and back (smiling). The zygomaticus major is perhaps the most noticeable. Sitting between the corners of our lips and the upper part of the cheeks, it controls the way in which we smile. The zygomaticus minor muscle is blending with fibers of the orbicularis oris (lips). Both muscles originate from the Zygomatic bone (cheek) and their insertion is the skin of the upper lip, and their nerve is the Facial Nerve and the Buccal branch. When there are trigger points in the zygomaticus muscles, they can cause pain up the cheek and along the side of the nose, past the medial corner of the eye and the eyebrows and in some cases in the middle of the forehead.

For bonuses go to ...

- **The Masseter Muscles:** The masseter muscles are the most prominent chewing muscles and responsible for the Temporomandibular joints pain (TMJ). The function is to elevate the mandible and close the jaw, the deep fiber is retruding the mandible. The trigger point pain in the *upper part* of the masseter muscle refers to the upper molars and maxilla, which is often described as Sinusitis. The trigger points in the *lower portion* of the masseter muscles refer to the lower molars and temple. All trigger points can cause tooth sensitivity.

In addition, the Masseter muscle commonly harbors trigger points and can get very tight with Bruxism (grinding teeth at night), along with the two Pterygoid muscles. The masseter muscle's origin is in the Zygomatic arch and Maxilla, and its insertion is the Coronoid Process and Ramus of mandible, and its Nerve is the Mandibular nerve.

Techniques: Other muscles to check before treating the masseter muscle are the Temporalis muscles, Pterygoids muscles, all face and neck muscles. Best manual therapy suggestion is to lay the client in a supine position, or if you decide to work intraoral (inside the mouth) palpate and examine these muscles: Levator Veli Palatini, Tensor Veli Palatini and Palatine Aponeurosis. These muscles are involved in the cause of chronic ear infection, as they play a role in keeping the Eustachian tube open. Use gentle to moderate pressure (it's a very sensitive area), use petrissage strokes downward and trigger point technique and hold tender's spots until release is felt.

- **Pterygoid Muscles Group:** The pterygoid muscles are two of the four muscles of mastication, located in the infratemporal fossa of the skull. These muscles are: lateral pterygoid and medial pterygoid. The primary function of the pterygoid muscles is to produce movements of the mandible at the temporomandibular joint, acting in grinding motion. Techniques: other muscles to examine and check are the masseter muscle, the temporalis, all facial muscles and neck muscles. NOTE: Pterygoid muscle groups are often key factors in pain in jaw, face, and ears. And they are a major player in the TMJ syndrome.

The origin of the lateral Pterygoid muscle is from the greater wing of the sphenoid and the pterygoid plate. Its insertion is the Condyloid process of the mandible and its nerve is from the mandible nerve. When there are trigger points in the lateral Pterygoid muscle it can cause pain in the temporal mandibular and maxillary sinus. NOTE: when this muscle hurts do not refer into the teeth, but in front of the ear and the cheek.

The origin of the medial Pterygoid muscle originates from the lateral pterygoid plate, palatine bone and the maxillary tuberosity. When there are trigger points in the medial Pterygoid muscle it can project vaguely into the back of the mouth and pharynx, and deep into the ear on the same side. Its insertion is an angle of the mandible, and its nerve is the mandibular nerve.

- **The Sternocleidomastoid Muscle (SCM):** The sternocleidomastoid muscle (SCM) is an important landmark in the neck which divides it into an anterior and a posterior triangle. It is a two-headed muscle: the sternal head and the clavicular head. Action of this muscle is to rotate the face to the opposite side and lift it towards the ceiling. Together the muscles flex the head and neck.

  The origin of the SCM is the Manubrium and medical clavicle. The insertion is the Mastoid process of the Temporal bone and superior Nuchal line. The Motor Nerve is Accessory Nerve, and the Sensory Nerve is the Cervical Plexus.

  The sternal head is more anterior, medial, and superficial. When there is trigger point pain in the sternal (superficial division) refers to the cheek and the supraorbital ridge. The highest points of pain refer to the occipital ridge and vertex of the head.

  The clavicular head is more posterior, lateral and deep. The lowest points of the clavicular head refer down into the sternum. When there are trigger points in the clavicular head, they can cause pain in the ribs (costal deep) and the forehead. The most superior or intense trigger point refers to the ear and can cause postural dizziness.

  NOTE: The SCM also maintains posture by helping to compensate for tilting of the shoulder girdle.

  Manual therapy suggestion is to lay the client in a supine position and use moderate pressure, stripping stroke downward, and trigger points technique until you feel a release. Use gentle effleurage and stretch the SCM afterwards. Other muscles to check are the Trapezius and chest muscles.

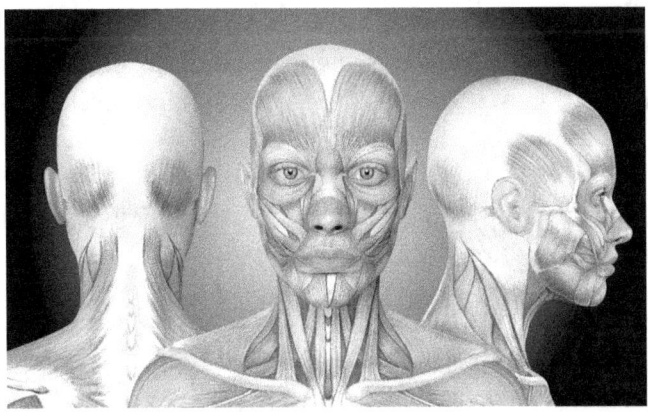

THE NECK

Muscles responsible for neck pain: *scalenes, sternocleidomastoid (already defined above), Trapezius muscle, Semispinalis Capitis Muscle, Splenius Capitis & Splenius Cervicis muscles, Levator Scapulae muscle*

- **The Scalene Muscle**: its action is to make lateral flexion in the neck and to help raise the ribs as an inappropriate accessory muscle in a paradoxical breathing. When there is pain in this muscle the trigger points can refer to two finger-like projections into the chest. Other common patterns of pain are into the shoulder, scapula and down the lateral arm, into the thumb and index finger. In addition, the Scalene muscle can impinge on the Brachial plexus, causing nerve pain and numbness down the arm. This is called Thoracic Outlet Syndrome.

Its origin of this muscle is C3-C6, and its insertion is the first or second rib. The scalene Minimus inserts into the Pleural dome. Its nerve is the Ventral Rami of the C3-C8 spinal nerves

Manual therapy suggestions: you can work in a supine, prone or seating position. Use a stripping stroke downward, a deep compression and friction on the clavicle and sternum areas. Be gentle because these areas are very sensitive. NOTE: when the neck pain is chronic, please check the muscles of the rotator cuff, anterior chest, and the arm.

- **Trapezius Muscle Group (Upper Fiber /Middle Fiber /Lower Fiber)**: This muscle group is part of the Posterior Neck muscles, and they are frequently in a state of constant straining due to poor posture, desk jobs, computer work, reading, and the extensive holding of a cell phone.

The function of the trapezius is to stabilize and move the scapula. The upper fibers can elevate and upwardly rotate the scapula and extend the neck. The middle fibers adduct (retract) the scapula. The lower fibers depress and aid the upper fibers in upwardly rotating the scapula. The points of origin for the middle and lower fibers are the posterior neck and shoulder and for the upper fiber is the Nuchal

Ligament and C6-T12 (Spinous Processes). This muscle group insertion is the Scapular Spine, Acromion process and distal clavicle. Their nerves are Accessory nerve (motor); Cervical Spinal nerves and C3 and C4 (motor and sensory).

When there are trigger points in the Trapezius muscle it can cause pain on the outer surface of the arm, proximal to the elbow. NOTE: This muscle group gets the most trigger points in the human body, causing common headaches.

- **Semispinalis Capitis Muscle**: its action is to do head extensions and assist with the head bending and rotations (side to side motion). When there are trigger points in this muscle it can cause pain into the temple area, with spillover into the lateral head. NOTE: This muscle can be a contributor to headaches. Its origin is in the Transverse process of lower cervical and upper thoracic vertebrae. Its insertion is in the area between superior and inferior nuchal line and its nerve is the Greater Occipital Nerve.

- **Splenius Capitis & Splenius Cervicis Muscles**: The bilateral action of these muscles helps with the head extensions and when there is a unilateral action it can rotate the head into the same side. When there are trigger points in these muscles they can cause pain in the vertex of the head, which can contribute to headaches. Other muscles to check when there is pain in this muscle are: the Levator Scapulae muscle, Serratus Posterior Superior Muscle and the deeper layers of the Multifidi and the Rotators' muscles.

For bonuses go to ...

Their origin is in the Ligamentum Nuchae, Spinous process of C7-T6. Their insertion is at the Occipital bone and the Mastoid process of the temporal bone, and their nerves are located at the C3 & C4.

Recommendations: Please learn more in detail about this group of soft tissue called Erector Spinae. NOTE: I will cover the Erector Spinae muscle group when we talk about the back.

- **Levator Scapulae Muscle**: NOTE: After the trapezius muscle, the Levator Scapulae muscle is the second most common muscle (region) that causes pain and tightness in the side of the neck and deep into the shoulders. Some of the reasons are the use of a heavy backpack or a heavy purse.

    The action of this muscle is to elevate the scapula and rotate the glenoid fossa downward. At the cervical attachment, it rotates the neck to the same side and assists extension. When this muscle is tight its main action is to restrict neck rotation "the classic stiff neck." NOTE: When in a forward head position, this muscle is often stretched and overworked. To help release this muscle you must put the head back by releasing the anterior chest and neck musculature.

    Its origin is at the Posterior Tubercles of the Transverse processes of C1-C4, and its insertion is at the Superior part of the medial border of the scapula. Its nerves are the Cervical nerve, C3-C4 and the dorsal Scapular nerve C5.

Manual therapy suggestion is to lay the client in a prone position and use heat and tens units on the back to reduce some of the tension in these areas before performing any treatment. Remember not to go over the client's pain tolerance limits. You can use the following modalities and techniques to release the pain: stripping strokes downward, petrissage, deep tissue massage, trigger point technique and pincer compression.

THE SHOULDER

The shoulder is made up of three bones: the scapula (shoulder blade), clavicle (collarbone) and humerus (upper arm bone). Two joints in the shoulder allow it to move: the acromioclavicular joint, where the highest point of the scapula (acromion) meets the clavicle, and the glenohumeral joint.

The muscles of the shoulder, chest and upper back are grouped in physical proximity with each other, mainly because the chest and the upper body control and influence the shoulder movements. Please note the rib muscles are not part of the shoulders but their function is more for respiration. The shoulders are divided by anterior and posterior shoulder muscles.

The scapula or shoulder blade is one of the most important structures of the shoulder because it functions as an anchor for the soft tissue muscles (The Rotator Cuff) and bones around the shoulders. The large area of the scapula has two bony areas called Ridge, which is in the spine superior and where the scapula attaches the muscles of the shoulders.

The spine of the scapula extends beyond the portion of the Acromion process and together with the clavicle they form the Acromioclavicular joint. They also form the hood where the head of the humerus bone is located, called the glenoid fossa. This connection creates the glenohumeral joint and structurally speaking this joint is very shallow.

The shoulders include the arms, and the arms are supported by various soft tissue muscles giving the shoulders and the arms freedom of movement. One of the many reasons why the shoulders are so vulnerable to injuries.
Since the scapula provides the socket of the arms it must move freely in every direction. The six muscles that hold the scapula in position during movement in different directions are: Pectoralis minor, Rhomboid major and minor, Levator Scapulae, Trapezius, and Serratus Anterior. Three other muscles which are very strong mover of the humerus are the Deltoid muscle, Pectoralis Major, and Latissimus Dorsi muscle. (I will discuss these muscles in detail later.)

NOTE: the scapulae is not joined into the back. The Collarbone (Clavicle) which it attaches to the shoulders by the Sternoclavicular joints has its own muscle, the Subclavius. (I will talk about this muscle in detail later in the book.
Muscles of the Anterior Shoulder are: the Subclavius Muscle, Pectoralis Major and Pectoralis Minor. NOTE: These muscles are also known as Chest Muscles.

- **The Subclavius Muscle**: Its origin is in the first rib cartilage and its insertion is in the inferior surface of the acromial, end of the clavicle. Its nerves are in the C5-C6 Cervical nerve branches and the Subclavian nerve. Its action is to fix the clavicle, elevate the first rib, and help protract the scapula by drawing the shoulders down and forward.

When there are trigger points in the Subclavius muscle it can cause pain toward the clavicle, over the shoulder, upper arm, radial side of the forearm, into the thumb and the first two fingers. If pain continues check these muscles: the Pectoralis major and minor and the Scalenes muscle.

Manual therapy suggestions: Lay the client in a supine (seated) position. Use gentle friction on the attachments of the inferior clavicle and the head humerus. Use the trigger point technique until the pain releases.

- **The Pectoralis Major**

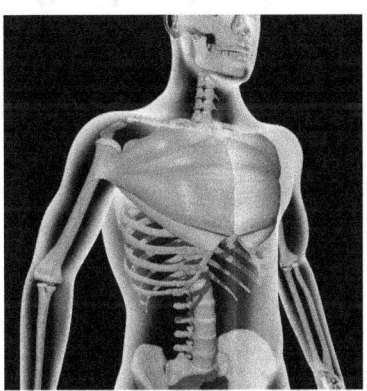

Is a thick, fan-shaped or triangular convergent muscle, situated at the chest of the human body. It makes up the bulk of the chest muscles and lies under the breast. Beneath the pectoralis major is the pectoralis minor, a thin, triangular muscle. Its origin is in the clavicular, the sternal, the costal parts, the anterior manubrium of the sternum, and the cartilages of the first to the sixth ribs, abdominal part to the aponeurosis of the **external oblique**. Its insertion is in the groove of the humerus to the lateral bicipital groove and its nerves are in the clavicle head, section C5-C6 and the sternocostal head, section C7-T1.

The pectoralis major extends across the upper part of the chest and is attached to a ridge at the rear of the humerus (the bone of the upper arm). Its major actions are adduction, or depression, of the arm (in opposition to the action of the deltoideus muscle) and rotation of the arm forward about the axis of the body.

The pectoralis major has three sections: clavicle, sternal, and coastal. Each of these sections runs in different directions to cross the sternoclavicular joint, the acromioclavicular, and the glenohumeral joint. Note: the pectoralis major fibers run to the abdominal aponeurosis.

When there are trigger points in the pectoralis major muscle it can cause pain on the clavicle section to the anterior shoulder, the sternal section down to the volar (referring to the palm of the hand), forearm, elbows, into the middle and ring fingers, and the costal and abdomen section transfer pain to the breast and nipples area. If the pain continues, check these muscles: Pectoralis Minor, the scalenes, sternocleidomastoid muscle (SCM), Sternalis, Subclavius, deltoids, biceps brachii, and Coracobrachialis.

Note: the trigger points in the left pectoralis major can mimic heart pain. Its most common dysfunction is the head-forward posture and also when this muscle is pulled the shoulders blades forward it can cause round shoulders. Rounded shoulders, sometimes known as "mom posture," are part of overall bad posture, and they can get worse if left untreated.

Manual therapy suggestions are: NOTE: Ask consent and permission from the clients (especially female clients) before treating this delicate and intimate area.

Lay the client in a supine position. Use heat or cold to increase circulation and induce relaxation and reduce tension before the treatment. Apply moderate to deep pressure, pincer compression and do friction on the attachments of the muscle stripping and sliding diagonally. Use of trigger point technique until the pain releases. NOTE: Remember to get feedback (from time to time) from the client while working in this sensitive area.

- **The Pectoralis Minor Muscle:** its action is to anchor the scapula to the chest and to draw the scapula forward, downward, and inward. Its origin is in the third to fifth ribs (near the costal cartilages). Its insertion is in the coracoid process of the scapula, and its nerve is in the Medial pectoral nerve, C8-T1.

NOTE: due to this muscle's function and actions during movement it is very susceptible to injuries.

When the pectoralis minor has trigger points pain it can cause pain to the arm and all the way down to the fingertips. NOTE: The bundle of nerves leading to the arm and the finger are called Brachial Plexus, which passes through the pectoralis minor, and it can entrap the brachial plexus causing numbness and weakness to the arm, hands, and fingers. If the pain continues check these muscles: the pectoralis major, scalene, SCM and all the Rotator cuff muscles.

Caution: to work and treat a client around the axilla or the armpit areas because major blood vessels and nerves are located there. Note: pain in the pectoralis minor is often associated by pain in the upper back muscles especially the Rhomboids. Also, the trigger point on the left side can mimic **angina (is chest pain caused by reduced blood flow to the heart muscles, heart attack or stroke).**

Manual therapy suggestions: Lay the client in a supine or side position. Use heat or ice treatment to induce relaxation in this sensitive area. Apply gentle to moderate pressure. Use stripping strokes, petrissage strokes, compression, and trigger point technique until the pain releases. Do gentle stretches on the neck and the shoulders after treatment. NOTE: Once again, be very careful of working around the armpit.

The posterior shoulder muscles are Supraspinatus Muscle, Infraspinatus Muscle, Teres Minor Muscle and the Subscapularis Muscle. NOTE: Also known as THE ROTATOR CUFF MUSCLES (SITS).

NOTE: although the Trapezius muscle is a neck muscle, it covers a vast territory of the upper back by covering the posterior shoulders and it plays an important role in moving and stabilizing the shoulders.

Muscles responsible for shoulder pain are: *Rotator Cuff muscles, Rhomboids major and minor muscles, and Serratus posterior superior muscle.*

- **The Supraspinatus Muscles (SITS)**: Their job is to stabilize the glenohumeral joint, in other words it has the control to internally rotate and lift the arm. NOTE: these muscle groups are small, and they demand together with the deltoid muscle in the abduction of the arm. For example: holding a heavy object or working with the arms raised (massage therapists have issues often with this muscle) or using a computer mouse for an extended period of time will also affect this muscle.

    When there are trigger points in the rotator cuff muscle it can cause pain and deep ache at the mid-deltoid area, and it could spillover down to the arm and the elbow.

    Its origin is in the Supraspinous fossa of the scapula and its insertion is in the Superior Facet of greater tubercle of the humerus. Its nerve is the Suprascapular nerve.

- **Infraspinatus Muscle**: its action is to externally rotate the humerus and to help stabilize the head of the humerus in the glenoid cavity during an upward movement of the arm. Its origin is in the Infraspinous fossa of the scapula, and its insertion is in the middle facet of the greater tubercle of the humerus. Its nerve is the Suprascapular nerve. NOTE:

in other words, this muscle allows you to externally rotate your arm at the shoulder socket.

When there are trigger points in the Infraspinatus muscle it can cause deep pain into the anterior shoulder joint, and it could spill over, down to the anterior arm. NOTE: Less common trigger points are near the lower medial border into the Rhomboids muscles.

- **Teres Minor Muscle:** this muscle functions as the little brother to the infraspinatus muscle, assisting it with an external rotation of the head of the humerus. NOTE: In other words, it is a small muscle that helps rotate your arm. Its origin is in the Lateral border of the scapula and its insertion is in the inferior facet of the greater tubercle of the humerus. Its nerve is the axillary nerve.

When there are trigger points in the Teres minor muscle it can cause pain that travels into the posterior deltoid and down to the posterior arm.

- **Subscapularis Muscle:** The origin of this muscle is at the Subscapular fossa and its insertion is at the Lesser tubercle of the humerus. Its nerves are the Upper & Lower Subscapular nerve (C5&C6).

Its action is to internally rotate the head of the humerus and adduct it. This muscle is in the medial rotator of the shoulder and is used to stabilize the shoulder. NOTE: by this adducting action it helps to keep the head of the humerus in the glenoid fossa. It's when a client complains that he/she is not able to raise the arm fully overhead (frozen shoulders).

When there are trigger points in the Subscapularis muscle it can cause pain primarily in the posterior shoulder and the pain can spillover into the posterior and medial arm and both sides of the wrist. If the pain is manifesting as a chronic and stabbing pain in the shoulder areas, check the trigger points in these muscles: the Latissimus Dorsi and Teres Major muscle. NOTE: Remember that these muscles also affect the upper back areas, mimicking deep pain between the shoulder blades, "the scapula." Keep in mind that this group of Rotator Cuff muscles have to do with the function and movement of the arm, hand and finger pain.

Manual therapy suggestions: Lay the client in a prone position, use heat and tens units on the tendered spots to reduce the tension and increase the circulation in the area. The trigger point techniques are: deep tissue, compression, friction, and pinched compression. You can also use an effleurage modality to relax the client after treatment.

- **Rhomboids Major and Minor Muscles**: the action of this muscle group is to retract, adduct, and draw the scapula in a medial position by using the lower fibers to rotate the scapula and turning the glenohumeral joint downward. NOTE: These muscles also prevent Scapular Winging.

    Their origin is in the Spinous processes of the T2-T5, and their insertion is in the medial border of the scapula. Their nerve is the Dorsal Scapular nerve, C4-C5.

    NOTE: When there are trigger points in the Rhomboids muscles the pain can be at the upper back pain, but it **is**

not a back issue, but rather a shoulder issue because these muscles are responsible to move the shoulders. The pain in the upper back is in the scapula because when the scapula rotates to lower the glenohumeral joint it forces the chest muscles, by pulling the shoulders forward and tightening the pectoral muscles.

- **Serratus Posterior Superior Muscle**

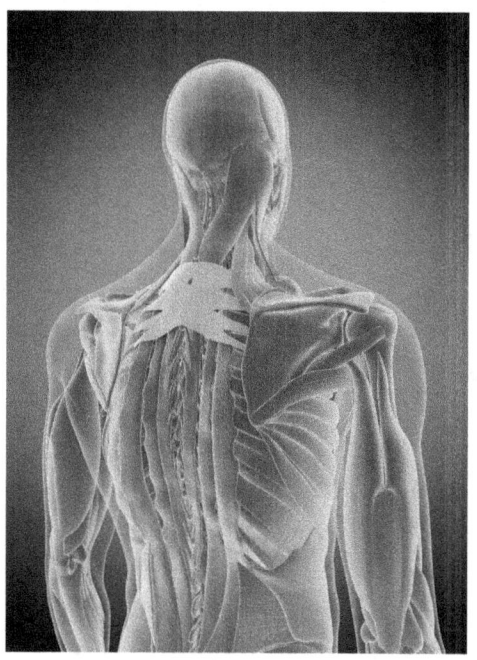

NOTE: some massage therapists may not know this muscle very well and they could consider it a mystery.

Its action is to elevate the ribs during inspiration (inhalation). Its origin is in the Nuchal Ligament, C7-T3 and the spinous processes. Its insertion is in the second to the fifth rib. Its nerve is the Intercostal nerve.

When there are trigger points in the Serratus posterior superior muscle it can cause pain and deep ache under the upper portion of the scapula. Sometimes the pain can spillover to the pectoral region. NOTE: very rarely the pain can extend to the shoulder, down to the arm, and to the little finger.

Manual therapy suggestions: NOTE: this area is very difficult to release the trigger points. Have the client in a prone position. Use heat and a tens unit in the entire shoulder, upper back, and posterior deltoid to increase circulation. The heat will relax the muscle and allow you to reach deeper layers. You can use these modalities: Stripping, petrissage, trigger point technique until you feel a release. Stretch the client after the treatment.

TORSO

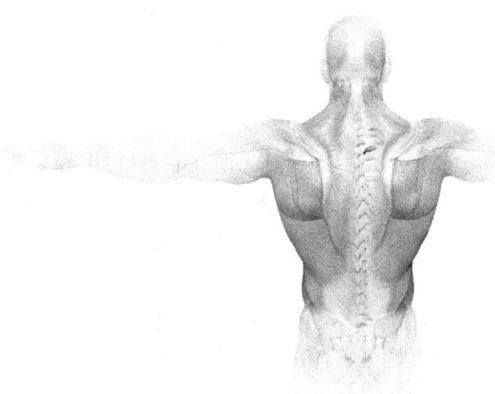

Muscles of the Thoracic region that causes pain are:
Latissimus Dorsi muscle, Serratus anterior muscle, Serratus posterior inferior Muscle, Deltoid Lateral and Anterior muscle group, Biceps Brachii Muscle, Brachialis muscle, Brachioradialis Muscle, Triceps Muscle group, The Anconeous Muscle.

- **The Latissimus Dorsi Muscle**: NOTE: this is a very large, broad, and powerful muscle that is hardly ever injured, but activities such as paddling a canoe or doing pull-ups at the gym will aggravate this giant.

    Its origin is in the Spinous processes of the thoracic T7-T12, thoracolumbar fascia, iliac crest and inferior 3 & 4 rib and the inferior angle of scapula. NOTE: In other words, this muscle, anatomically speaking, takes the anterior aspect of the arm, anchoring the arm to the lower back and the pelvis; plus it is near the Teres Major, and together they bundle the posterior border of the axilla.

    Its action is to adduct and internally rotate the arm at the shoulder and the forceful depression of the scapula. Its insertion is the floor of the intertubercular groove of the humerus and its nerves are the Thoracodorsal nerves C6-C8.

    When there are trigger points in this muscle the pain and discomfort can be over the inferior angle of the scapula into the armpit area, down to the back of the arm and into the last two fingers. The pain can spill over, down the posterior arm and hand. If so, check the trigger points in these muscles: Serratus posterior inferior, Serratus anterior, pectoralis minor, pectoralis interior, and exterior obliques. Also, an unusual trigger point in the anterior mid muscle can cause pain into the anterior shoulder. NOTE: These muscles are frequently overlooked and very few massage therapists work on them or even know how they function.

Manual therapy suggestions are: lay the client in a sideway or prone position. Use heat or a tens unit and use moderate to deep pressure. You can use these modalities: trigger point technique, pinch compression and an effleurage in the entire back, including the posterior arm and the neck.

- **Serratus Anterior Muscle**: NOTE: this muscle is located on the side of the chest and it's worth to mention under the TORSO MUSCLES category because its action is the rotation of the scapula to turn the glenoid fossa upward, protraction and elevation of the scapula and prevention of winging of the scapula.

Its origin is the fleshy slips from the outer surface of the upper 8 & 9 rib and its insertion is in the medial margin of the scapula. Its nerve is the Long Thoracic nerve (roots of the Brachial Plexus C5-C7).

This muscle works with the pectoral muscles and opposes the Rhomboids muscles' actions, so when there are trigger points in this muscle it can cause pain in the side of the chest and down to the arm. NOTE: it mimics the pectoralis minor trigger point pain because of its attachments to the 1st to the 8th ribs, which elevate and rotate the scapula.

The muscle fibers are in a diagonal position. NOTE: Remember to apply moderate pressure moderately because this muscle is extremely sensitive.

- **Serratus Posterior Inferior Muscle**: its action is to depress the lower ribs, assist with the rotation and extension of the trunk (torso area) and respiration. The origin of this muscle is at the medial inferior of the Latissimus Dorsi muscle, the second vertebrae of the lower thoracic, the third upper lumbar vertebrae, and the last four ribs. Its insertions are at the 9th-12th ribs, and its nerve is the intercostal nerves, T9-T12. NOTE: this muscle is definitely a troublemaker for the lower back.

When there are trigger points in the Serratus posterior inferior muscle, they can cause pain across the back and over the lower ribs. If the pain continues you can check trigger points for these muscles: Quadratus Lumborum (QL), Iliocostalis thoracis, Psoas major, Rectus abdominis, Pyramidalis and the Diaphragm.

NOTE: To avoid any more problems with this powerful group of Serratus muscles, it's essential to learn breathing techniques through the diaphragm.

Diaphragmatic breathing, or "belly breathing," involves fully engaging the stomach, abdominal muscles, and diaphragm when breathing. This means actively pulling the diaphragm down with each inward breath. In this way, diaphragmatic breathing helps the lungs fill more efficiently.

- **Deltoid Lateral, Anterior, and Posterior Muscle Group**: as a whole the deltoid laterally abducts the humerus at the glenohumeral joint. The anterior deltoid forward flexes the arms, as well as horizontally flexing the arm across the chest. NOTE: The attachment of the anterior portion of this muscle looks like it should medially rotate the arm, but this has been disproved by electromyography studies.

   The origin of this muscle group is the clavicle, acromion and the spine of the scapula. Its insertion is the deltoid tuberosity of the humerus, and its nerve is the axillary nerve.

   When there are trigger points in the anterior deltoid muscle, they can cause pain in the anterior and lateral of the shoulder. For the posterior deltoid the trigger points can cause pain in the posterior part of the shoulder, and it could spill over, down to the lateral arm. NOTE: the deltoid muscle group is prompt to trigger points. If the client is still in pain, check these muscles for trigger points: the rotator cuff muscles (especially the Infraspinatus), the teres major, and the pectoralis major.

   Manual therapy suggestions: have the client lie down in a supine position. Use heat at the top of the chest and shoulders. Apply moderate to deep pressure and use trigger point techniques until the muscle releases. I recommend passively stretching the client after treatment.

- **Biceps Brachii Muscle**: the biceps are attached to the radius. It helps to flex the elbow and move the forearm into supinate position. NOTE: you can test this by watching your biceps get shorter as you turn your palm up.

Its origin is in the short-head coracoid process of the scapula and the long-head of the supraglenoid tubercle. Its insertion is in the radial tuberosity and the bicipital aponeurosis, deep into the fascia on the medial part of the forearm. Its nerve is the musculocutaneous nerve (C5-C7).

When there are trigger points in the biceps Brachii muscle it can cause pain in the main referral pattern that is up into the shoulder, with spillover into the posterior aspect, above the scapula. NOTE: a less common trigger point is into the anterior elbow and forearm. The most common injury to this area is an inflamed upper biceps tendon. In mild cases, massage therapists can use the cross-fiber friction modality to reduce inflammation and stimulate healing.

- **Brachialis Muscle**: NOTE: By far, the Brachialis muscle is one of the most neglected muscles by most massage therapists.

Its origin is at the anterior surface of the humerus, particularly the distal half of this bone. Its insertion is at the Coronoid process and the tuberosity of the ulna. Its nerve is the Musculocutaneous nerve.

The brachialis is the strongest flexor of the elbow. It lies deep into the Biceps. NOTE: Unlike the Bicep, this muscle does not insert onto the Radius and therefore it cannot participate in a pronation/supination of the forearm.

When there are trigger points in the Brachialis muscle it can cause pain into the thumb, with secondary patterns into the anterior arm and the anterior elbow joint.

- **Brachioradialis Muscle**: its action is to flex the elbow. Its origin is in the Lateral supracondylar ridge of the humerus and its insertion is of the Distal radius. Its nerve is the Radial nerve.

When there are trigger points in the Brachioradialis muscle it can cause pain in the lateral elbow, forearm, and the thumb. If the pain continues, you can check for trigger points in these muscles: Supinator, Opponens pollicis, and Adductor pollicis.

NOTE: Some massage therapists forget that this muscle is an elbow flexor and that it lies over the forearm and is attached onto the Styloid process of the distal radius.

Manual therapy suggestions: lay the client in a supine position, use moderate to deep pressure (if possible), stripping upward and use a trigger point technique until it releases. I recommend a gentle stretch after the treatment.

- **Triceps Muscle Group:** NOTE: this is another popular muscle, the Triceps Brachii muscle.

The action of this muscle group is to extend the elbow. This muscle group have three heads: the long- head, which originates at the infraglenoid tubercle of the scapula. The Lateral-head, which originates at the posterior humerus, and the Medial-head, which originates also at the posterior humerus. The insertion of this muscle group is at the Olecranon process of ulna and the nerve is the Radial Nerve.

The Medial head is the deepest head of the triceps and is the workhorse of the three heads and it is the head that contracts first and with most (greater) force.

When there are trigger points in the long head of the triceps muscle it can cause pain into the posterior shoulder and sometimes down into the posterior forearm (skipping the elbow). The trigger points in the center of the medial head can cause pain into the Olecranon process (the elbow). NOTE: Trigger points in the lateral part of the medial head refer to the lateral Epicondyle and are a common component of "Tennis Elbow." If the client still has pain, you can check the trigger points in these muscles: all the arm muscles (posterior and anterior), the rotator cuff, and the pectoralis muscle (major and minor).

Manual therapy suggestions: lay the client in a supine or prone position and be very gentle when moving the arm back. Use moderate to deep pressure, do friction by the elbow, use petrissage or trigger point technique until it releases.

ARMS & FOREARM

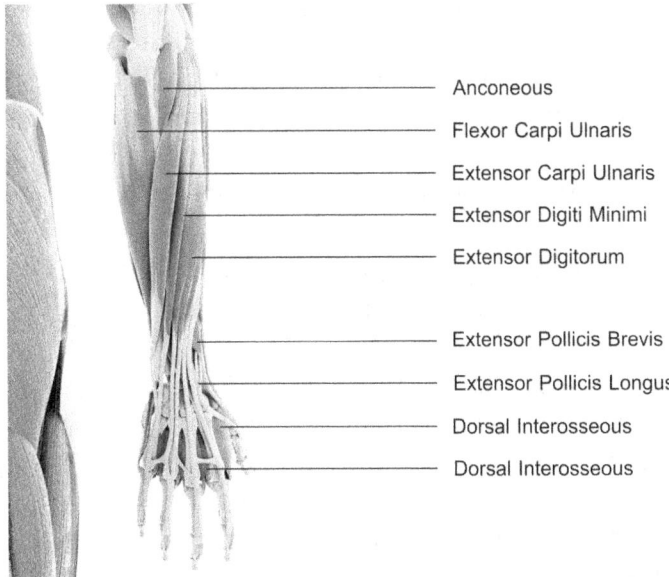

- Anconeous
- Flexor Carpi Ulnaris
- Extensor Carpi Ulnaris
- Extensor Digiti Minimi
- Extensor Digitorum
- Extensor Pollicis Brevis
- Extensor Pollicis Longus
- Dorsal Interosseous
- Dorsal Interosseous

The muscles of the arms and forearm that cause pain are: *Anconeous muscle, Coracobrachialis muscle, Supinator muscle, and Pronator Teres muscle.*

- **The Anconeous Muscle**: NOTE: in my opinion this muscle is also on the list of unknown and mysterious muscles for some massage therapists.

  The Anconeous muscle origin is in the Lateral Epicondyle of the humerus, and the insertion is the Lateral surface of the Olecranon process of the ulna and posterior ulna. Its nerve is the Radial nerve C7-T1.

Its action is to assist the Triceps with an elbow extension. This muscle assists abduction of the ulna during pronation of the hand and helps to stabilize the humeroulnar joint.

Where there are trigger points in the Anconeus muscle it can cause pain in the lateral Epicondyle. NOTE: The pain can also create tension on muscles like the Scalene, Supraspinatus and Serratus posterior superior.

Manual therapy suggestions: NOTE: The Anconeous is small and thin muscle. And is rarely injured.

Use moderate pressure, stripping, friction, and trigger point technique until the muscle releases. Applying static pressure to the muscle's belly with a fingerprint while flexing and extending the elbow. This modality is an effective and safe way to soften this muscle and release any trigger points.

- **The Coracobrachialis Muscle**: NOTE: this is another muscle that is not well known by massage therapists. The function of this muscle is to assist flexion and adduction of the humerus and to keep the head of the humerus in the glenoid fossa.

Its origin is at the coracoid process of the scapula and is a neighboring muscle to the biceps brachii and the pectoralis minor. Its insertion is at the medial humerus and its nerve is the Musculocutaneous nerve, C5-C7.

When there are trigger points in the Coracobrachialis muscle it can cause pain in the upper arm, forearm, mid and anterior deltoid, and the hand. If the pain continues, check these muscles: rotator cuff muscles, all the muscle of the arm and the deltoid.

Manual therapy suggestions: to reach this muscle, we have to work under the bicep and get close to the armpit. NOTE: Be careful with the axilla area and avoid nerve branches and blood vessels that pass under the coracoid process into the arm.

- **The Supinator Muscle**: this muscle is very deep and works along with the bicep's supinator function. Its origin is in the Lateral epicondyle of the humerus, supinator crest of ulna, radial collateral ligament, and the annular ligament. Its insertion is in the Lateral proximal radial shaft and its nerve is the Radial nerve.

  When there are trigger points in the Supinator muscle it can cause pain into the lateral aspect of the elbow with spillover into the dorsal part of the thumb and the index finger. If the pain continues, check these muscles for trigger points: Infraspinatus, Subclavius, Scalene, Brachialis, Anconeous, Brachioradialis and Extensor of the hand.

  Manual therapy suggestions: lay the client in a supine position and hold the arm in a pronation position (backwards or downward). Use a trigger points technique until you feel the release.

- **The Pronator Teres Muscle**: Its action is to assist the Pronator Quadratus muscle and the primary pronator, in fast movements and to overcome resistance and to flex the elbow.

Its origin is in the Humeral head, medial epicondyle of the humerus/ ulnar head at the coronoid process of the ulna. Its insertion is the Radius, and its nerve is the Medial nerve.

When there are trigger points in the Pronator Teres muscle it can cause deep into the wrist and the base of the thumb (anterior forearm). If the pain continues, check the trigger points in these muscles: Scalene, Infraspinatus and Subclavius.

Manual therapy suggestions: Lay the client in a supine position and expose the crease of the elbow. Then compress on the medial epicondyle. Do a gentle stretch after the treatment.

The next group of muscles is the extensor of the hand, wrist and fingers.

This group of muscles covers the dorsal part of the forearm and stabilize the wrist during the hand movement. These muscles are vital to the gripping motion because the wrist extends during the grip increasing the grip power. NOTE: This group of muscles is superficial and easy to treat, but massage therapists have issues working with this group of muscles.

Its job is to extend and abduct the wrist and the attachments of this muscle group are the lateral humerus and the distal to the third metacarpal.

Its origin is in the Lateral epicondyle of the humerus. Its insertion is in the base of the 3rd metacarpal and its nerve is the Radial nerve. When there are trigger points in these muscles it can cause pain on the dorsal surface of the hand. If the pain continues, check the trigger points in these muscles: Subscapularis, Infraspinatus, Coracobrachialis and the Brachialis muscle.

- **Extensor Carpi Radialis Longus Muscle:** This muscle extends and abducts the wrist. Its origin is in the Lateral supracondylar ridge of the humerus and its insertion is the base of the 2nd metacarpal. Its nerve is the radial nerve. When there are trigger points in the Extensor Carpi Radialis Longus muscle it can cause pain primarily to the lateral epicondyle and secondarily, in the anatomical snuff box-between the thumb and first finger. The pain can also spill over, down to the posterior arm, elbow, dorsal hand, and the forearm.

- **Extensor Carpi Ulnaris Muscle:** Extensor Carpi Ulnaris muscle's role is to extend and deviate to the wrist (Ulnar Deviation). Its origin is the Lateral Epicondyle of the humerus and the posterior ulna. Its insertion is the base of the 5th metacarpal, and its nerve is the Radial nerve.

  When there are trigger points in the Extensor Carpi Ulnaris muscle it can cause pain into the posterior ulnar side of the wrist. If the pain continues, check the trigger points for these muscles: the Coracobrachialis and the Subclavius muscles.

NOTE: The Extensor Carpi Ulnaris muscle harbors trigger points less often than the Exterior Carpi Radialis Brevis muscle and the Longus.

- **Abductor Minimi Digiti Muscle:** Its action is to abduct the little finger. NOTE: This muscle is actually half of what would be the next dorsal interosseus muscle if the fingers continued. Its origin is in the Pisiform and its insertion in the base of the small finger proximal phalanx. Its nerve is the Ulnar nerve.

  When there are trigger points in the Abductor Minimi Digiti muscle it can cause pain in the little finger. NOTE: Like the interosseous muscles of the hand, this muscle refers to the finger that it controls.

- **Extensor Digitorum:** Its action is to extend the fingers and to assist the wrist extension. Its origin is in the lateral epicondyle of the humerus, and its insertion is the extensor expansion of the digits 2-5. Its nerve is the radial nerve.

  When there are trigger points in the Extensor Digitorum it can cause pain into the middle or second finger. The pain can spillover down to the dorsal aspect of the arm. NOTE: Trigger points in the middle finger are the most common. Also, if there are trigger points in the ring finger extensor the pain can go into the lateral epicondyle.

- **Extensor Indicis Muscle:** Its action is to extend the index finger and once the fingers are fully extended, this muscle can also help extend the wrist. Its origin is in the Posterior ulna and the interosseous membrane. Its insertion is in the extensor hood expansion of the index finger and its nerve is the Posterior Interosseus nerve.

When there are trigger points in the Extensor Indicis muscle it can cause pain in the posterior wrist and the hand. NOTE: The pain does not reach into the index finger or the little finger because these fingers have separate extensors, and they move independently from other fingers.

- **Extensor Pollicis Brevis Muscle:** Its action is to extend and abduct the thumb. NOTE: The extensor pollicis brevis (EPB) belongs to the deep group of the posterior fascial compartment of the forearm. It is a part of the lateral border of the anatomical snuffbox, also known as the radial fossa.

When there are trigger points in the Extensor Pollicis Brevis muscle it can cause pain in the thumb, but the pain can spill over to the Subscapularis and the Serratus posterior superior.

Manual therapy suggestions: The modalities and treatment for these extensor muscles are done as a group, all these muscles get treated together. Use stripping compression, petrissage, or friction into the attachments and trigger points techniques until the muscles release. Use passive stretches after treatment.

WRIST

The wrist is also called carpus with a complex joint between the five metacarpal bones of the hand, the radius, and the ulna bones of the forearm. The wrist is composed of eight or nine small, short bones (carpal bones) roughly arranged in two rows. Their tendons pass through the carpal tunnel and when stiffness and swelling can trap the median nerve, causing carpal tunnel syndrome.

NOTE: massage therapists suffer from carpal tunnel syndrome for the extensive and excessive use of their hands. One way to improve this condition is by relaxing the flexor muscles in the forearm.

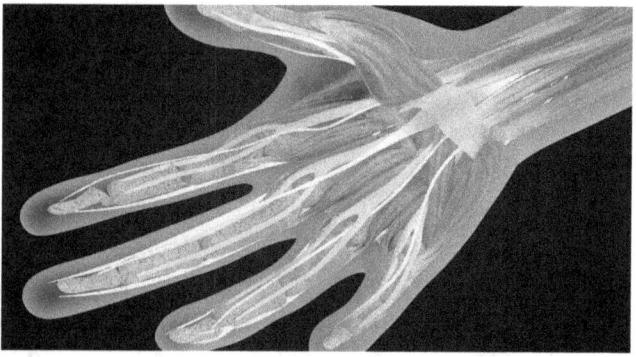

Muscles of the Wrist

- **The Flexor Retinaculum**: (aka Transverse Carpal Ligament) is located between the hamate, pisiform, and the trapezium bones. Manual therapy suggestions: Use friction and deep massage on the palmar surface of the hand.

- **Palmaris Longus Muscle:** Its origin is on top of the flexor retinaculum, and it is a small muscle in the medial humerus and stretches to the palm.

  Its action is to cuff the hand and to flex the wrist. When there are trigger points in the Palmaris Longus muscle it can cause pain like a pricking-needle sensation. If the pain continues, check the trigger points in these muscles: the Vola surface of the forearm, all the flexors of the forearm, the pronator teres, the Serratus anterior, and the pectoralis.

- **The Flexor Carpi Radialis:** its action is to flex and radially deviate the wrist. NOTE: this muscle is one of the three main wrist flexors. Its origin is in the medial epicondyle of the humerus and its insertion is in the base of the 2nd and the 3rd metacarpals. Its nerve is the Median nerve.

  When there are trigger points in the Flexor Carpi Radialis muscle it can cause pain into the wrist. If the pain continues, check the trigger points of the pronator teres muscles. NOTE: The trigger points can mimic the wrist pain associated with Carpal Tunnel Syndrome, except the finger numbness or pain.

- **The Flexor Carpi Ulnaris:** Its action is to flex and ulnar deviate the wrist. Its origin is in the Ulnar head-olecranon & posterior ulnar and also in the humeral head-medial epicondyle of the humerus.

  Its insertions are the Pisiform, hamate, and the 5th metacarpal base. Its nerve is the Ulnar nerve.

When there are trigger points in the Flexor Carpi Ulnaris muscle it can cause pain in the Ulnar side of the wrist. If the pain continues, check the trigger points of these muscles: the pectoralis muscles and the Serratus posterior superior muscles.

The Flexor Digitorum: Superficialis & Profundus Muscles

- **The Flexor Digitorum Superficialis**: flexes the middle phalanges of the medial four digits at the proximal interphalangeal joints. It also flexes the proximal phalanges at the metacarpophalangeal joints and the wrist joint. Flexor digitorum superficialis can flex each finger it serves independently. Its origin is at the Medial Epicondyle of the humerus, as well as the radius and ulna. Its insertion is at the bases of the middle phalanges of the four fingers and its nerve is the Median nerve.

- **The Flexor Digitorum Profundus**: lies deep to the superficialis, but it attaches more distally (Anatomically located far from a point of reference, such as an origin or a point of attachment). Therefore, profundus's tendons go through the tendons of superficialis, and end up attaching to the distal phalanx. For this reason, the profundus muscle is also called the perforating muscle.

When there are trigger points in the Flexor Digitorum Superficialis & Profundus muscles it can cause pain in the same digit that the muscle fibers activate. Applying deep pressure into the forearm while the client flexes and extends their fingers is an effective way to release the trigger points. NOTE: The Flexor Digitorum Superficialis and Profundus are the deepest muscles on the forearm, and both control the fingers. They are important because the attachments are in each finger.

- **The Flexor Pollicis Longus Muscle**: Its action is to flex the thumb and its origin is in the Radius and interosseous membrane. Its insertion is on the base of the distal thumb phalanx and its nerve is the medial nerve. When there are trigger points in the Flexor Pollicis Longus muscle it can cause pain into the thumb. Other muscles to check for trigger points are: the Scalene and the Subclavius muscles. NOTE: it's possible that the pain can travel to the anterior wrist but is not supported by research.

  Manual therapy suggestions: NOTE: This group of wrist muscles must be treated together. Lay the client in a supine position. Stabilize the arm and use these techniques: stripping, petrissage, compression, or trigger point technique until the muscles release. Use friction and then apply gentle stretches after treatment. NOTE: Do not forget to work on each finger individually.

Muscles of the Hand

- **The Thumb (first metacarpal)**: The thumb is the short and thick first or most preaxial digit of the human hand that differs from the other fingers in having only two phalanges, in having greater freedom of movement, and in being opposable to the other fingers. The ball of the thumb is the Thenar Eminence and its muscles are the Adductor

Pollicis, which has two heads. The attachments of the thumb go as far as the middle hand, which is attached to the second and the third metacarpal, the trapezoid, and the Capitate bone, which is close to the wrist. NOTE: Remember that the thumb has a separate join, the carpometacarpal.

Cover the primary troublemaker of the muscle of the hand: the thumb (first metacarpal). When the thumb hurts it can mimic the pain like carpal tunnel syndrome. When there are trigger points in this muscle it can cause pain in both sides of the thumb area. If the pain continues, check these muscles: Opponens pollicis, Supinator, Brachioradialis, Brachialis, Infraspinatus, Subclavius and the Scalene muscle. NOTE: Pain in the thumb can make compensations and dysfunction that travels from the forearm, the neck and the shoulder.

- **The Flexor Pollicis Brevis**: Its action is to raise the dorsal surface of the radius and extend the first phalanx of the thumb and adducts the hand. The Flexor Pollicis Brevis attaches the proximal to the trapezium, the flexor retinaculum of the wrist, the first metacarpal bone, and the distal to the base of the phalanx of the thumb.

Manual technique suggestion: use friction on the thenar eminence, pinching compression, and trigger point technique until it releases.

- **Abductor Pollicis Brevis**: This muscle is a thin flat muscle, and its action is to abduct the thumb by way of the metacarpophalangeal joint and the carpometacarpal joint.

In addition, it provides some assistance in the opposition and extension of the thumb.

- **Opponens Pollicis**: The Opponens pollicis is a small, triangular muscle in the hand, which functions to oppose the thumb. It is one of the three thenar muscles. It lies deep to the abductor pollicis brevis and the lateral to the flexor pollicis brevis.

When there are trigger points in the Opponens pollicis it can cause pain in the thumb (itself), the wrist, and in the head of the Radius. If the pain continues, you can check these muscles: adductor Pollicis, Infraspinatus, Brachialis, Subscapularis, Subclavius, scalene, Serratus anterior & posterior superior, and Coracobrachialis muscle.

Manual therapy suggestions: start the treatment with the palm up. Use a trigger points technique and friction on the wrist, until it releases. NOTE: work the whole hand and the fingers, including the interosseous muscles of the hand. Especially the ulnar (pinky) side of the hand.

Recommendation: We can apply the same manual therapy suggestions and modalities (trigger points technique and friction) to treat all the muscles of the hand because we can find similar issues/troubles in these muscles' attachments, which are in constant labor and do a lot of repetitive motion and movements

In addition, pain in the Flexor Digiti Minimi Brevis and Abductor Digiti Minimi are cases related to the triceps and the Latissimus Dorsi muscles, due to their trigger points in the ulnar side of the hand.

For bonuses go to ...

THE MUSCLES OF THE ABDOMINAL REGION, THE PELVIS, AND THE LOWER BACK/LUMBAR REGION

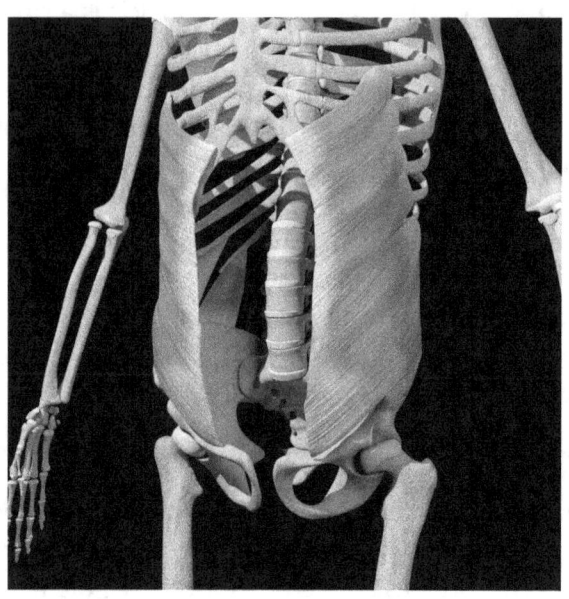

The abdominal region is also known as the belly, tummy, or stomach. The abdominal region is clinically important because the abdominal cavity houses important viral organs, major blood vessels, arteries, and nerves.

The abdominal muscles group is located between the thorax and the pelvic. Therefore, these muscles are associated with lower back pain. The muscles forming the abdomen wall are the Rectus Abdominis, Pyramidalis, Abdominal Obliques (External & Internal) and the transversus abdominis. All these muscles assist in exhalation while they're compressing the abdominal cavity.

When there are trigger points in Abdominal muscles they can cause pain into the viscera, causing problems like Somatovisceral disease. This disease is pertaining to the influence of the body framework (soma), or neuromusculoskeletal system and the function of the internal body systems and organs.

Muscles of the Abdomen

- **The Rectus Abdominis Muscle**: The Rectus Abdominis muscle is separated by the línea alba which means 'white line' in Latin. This muscle is a tendinous, fibrous raphe that runs vertically down the midline of the abdomen. It extends between the inferior limit of the xiphoid bone (sternum) and the pubis.

    Its action is to flex the lumbar column and to rotate the spine and it also increases the intra-abdominal pressure and resists the extension of the spine. Its origin is in the pubis and its insertions are into the xiphoid process and the fifth to seventh rib. Its nerve is the Thoracic abdominal nerve, T7-T12.

    When there are trigger points in the Rectus Abdominis muscle it can cause pain over the abdomen: from the xiphoid bone (sternum) to the pubis, across the back just below the scapulae (the region around the epigastrium and precordium). Then the pain goes to the top of the buttocks (iliac crest) and the sacrum into the lower lateral quadrant of the abdomen, mid-abdomen just inferior to the umbilicus, the abdominal fullness and the dysmenorrhea. If the pain continues, check these muscles for trigger points: the Pyramidalis muscle, Serratus posterior inferior, Iliopsoas, Abdominal Obliques, Transversus abdominis, Gluteal muscles and the Quadratus Lumborum (QL).

NOTE: The fact that this muscle refers to pain in the back, means that if you're working on the back Erector group and are not providing relief, then look for trigger points in the Rectus Abdominis muscle. This muscle will also be tightened in clients who slouch or have a posterior rotated pelvis. But if a client has an anterior rotated pelvis (which is most common) strengthening this muscle can help the hips come back into alignment. It's not true, however, that strengthening the Rectus Abdominis muscle will automatically help with the lower back pain.

Manual therapy suggestion: lay the client in a supine position. Use a proper draping to cover this part of the body and ask for consent if you're doing compressions by the pubis. Use heat or ice to induce circulation and to reduce tension. Use gentle to moderate pressure (because there are visceral organs under the abdomen). Use cross-fiber strokes and trigger point techniques until the pain releases. Finish the treatment with effleurage.

- **The Pyramidalis Muscle:** Its action is to tense the Linea Alba. Its origin is in the pubis symphysis and crest and its insertion is in the lower portion of the Linea Alba. Its nerve is the Subcostal nerve, T12.

When this muscle has a trigger point the pain can shift near the midline between the pubic bone to the umbilicus (belly button). If the pain continues, check the trigger points in these muscles: Rectus abdominis, Iliopsoas and Abdominal Obliques.

Manual therapy suggestions: lay the client in a supine position. Use proper draping to cover the client properly and ask for consent to work in this intimate area. Use gentle to moderate pressure and use compression and trigger point techniques until the pain releases.

NOTE: This muscle is absent in 20% of people: The pyramidalis muscle was present in 92% cases, usually bilaterally (72%) than unilaterally (20%) and more frequently in males (94.11%) than in females (87.5%).

- **Abdominal Obliques (External & Internal) Muscles:** The external & internal abdominal obliques are discernible only when contracted by raising one shoulder toward the opposite side of the body. These two-muscles run in the same direction as the intercostal muscles. As their name implies, the external & internal obliques' architecture speaks of their muscle fibers being parallel.

Their action is to flex and rotate the vertebral column. In other words, bilaterally, increase intra-abdominal pressure and flex the spine. Unilaterally, assist in lateral flexion and rotation of the spine. When the external oblique muscle develops pain it can run along the epigastric region, over the chest, below the costal arch, and up and down the abdomen region. NOTE: Upper trigger points can mimic a heartburn.

The origin of the external obliques is in the 5th to the 12th rib. Its insertion is in the inferiorly to the anterior half of the lateral iliac crest, the inguinal ligament, and the anterior layer of the rectus sheath. Its nerves are the lower 6th intercostal nerve and the subcostal nerve.

The origin for the internal oblique is in the inguinal ligament, iliac crest, and the Lumbodorsal fascia. Its insertion is in the Linea Alba, xiphoid process, and the inferior ribs. Its nerves are the Peripheral nerve (VPR) and the Segmental Nerve, T6-T12 & L1.

When there are trigger points in the internal oblique muscle it can cause pain in the lower quadrant of the abdomen. Also, the lower trigger points can spillover into the umbilicus, inguinal ligament, and the genitals. If the pain continues, check these muscles: Pyramidalis, Serratus posterior inferior, Iliopsoas, Gluteus muscles and Quadratus Lumborum (QL). NOTE: the variability in the research may be due to the difficulty isolating the different muscle layers and active trigger points can cause belching, heartburn, and diarrhea.

Manual therapy suggestions: lay the client in a supine position. Do a myofascial stretching and be incredibly careful not to harm any organs by using too much pressure. Use trigger point (gentle) compression, effleurage, and cross-fiber techniques until the pain releases.

- **Transversus Abdominis Muscle:** The transversus abdominis (TrA) muscle is the deepest of the 6 abdominal muscles. It extends between the ribs and the pelvis, wrapping around the trunk from front to back. The fibers of this muscle run horizontally, similar to a back support belt.

  Its action is to compress the abdomen. When there are trigger points in this muscle it can cause pain along and between the anterior costal margin. If the pain continues, check these muscles: the Rectus abdominis and the Abdominal Obliques.

  Note: this muscle lies deeper than the other abdominal muscles and they are not separate manual treatment for it, and it cannot be palpable.

THE PELVIS

You need client's consent when you treat and examine a client in these intimate and sensitive areas. Please approach the examination and the treatment with a great deal of respect, privacy, modesty, and professionalism. NOTE: The muscles of the pelvis should always be considered and addressed in any consult and assessment because they balance the torso and the appendages on the leg.

The muscles of the anterior pelvis are the Psoas Major (Iliopsoas) muscle, the Iliacus muscle, the Psoas Minor.

- **The Psoas (Iliopsoas) Muscle**: The psoas muscle's major job is to flex the hip and postural muscle. The origin of the Psoas muscle attaches to the lumbar vertebrae and passes downward through the abdominal cavity to the groin, where it merges with the Iliacus muscle and passes over the anterior rim of the Ilium muscle, then obliquely in a posterior and inferior direction to be attached to the Lesser Trochanter of the femur. In other words, this muscle is located on the vertebral bodies and disc of T12-L5, and the insertion is into the lesser trochanter of the femur and the nerve is Spinal nerve L2-L4. In addition, the psoas muscle (joints) attaches to the Iliacus muscle at the groin to form the Iliopsoas muscle. This muscle is considered the "filet mignon of the body" and it's especially important in the stability of walking and the hip flexibility. When the leg is fixed, the psoas extends the lumbar spine (increases the lumbar lordosis). NOTE: since we walk upright, much greater muscular effort is required to flex the hip and lift the leg.

Additionally, the Psoas muscle plays a major role in determining the positioning of the pelvis and the lower back in relation to each other. Also, most people spend more time in a sitting position therefore the Iliopsoas muscle spends a lot of time shortened and very little time stretched

NOTE: Due to bad posture and sitting for an extended period of time, this muscle shortens during pregnancy and holds the baby on the hip in extension. Because the psoas anatomical attachments affect the back, groin, and leg by the knee and when the pelvis is tilted forward create lordosis, when anterior pelvic rotation grinds the abdomen cavity forward and to protrude (swells)

When there are trigger points in the Psoas muscle it can cause pain primarily to the lower lumbar area and the sacrum and secondly to the anterior thigh. NOTE: Trigger points in the Psoas can mimic appendicitis. If the pain continues, check these muscles: Iliacus, Rectus Abdominis, Obliques, Diaphragm, Hip Adductors, the Quadratus Lumborum muscle (QL), the Erector spinae group.

Manual therapy suggestions: Lay the client in a supine position. Use heat on the abdomen and the quadriceps. Use trigger point technique until the pain releases and compression on attachments of the lesser trochanter.

Iliacus muscle is the neighbor of the Psoas. Treat it the same way and the pelvic floor muscles can fall in the category of contraindication, outside our scope of practice for massage therapists. Others can be treated of course with client consent and modesty.

- **The Iliacus Muscles**: this muscle works together with the Psoas muscle. Its action is to flex the hip and its origin is the iliac fossa. Its insertion is to the tendon of the Psoas muscle, the anterior surface of the trochanter, and the capsule of the hip joint. The nerve is L2-L3 spinal nerves. Trigger point pain is the same as the Psoas muscle.

- **The Psoas Minor Muscle**: Action assists in flexion of the lumbar spine. Its origin is superiorly to the 12th thoracic and the first Lumbar vertebrae and the disk between both of them. Its insertion is in the iliopectineal arch (iliac fascia). NOTE: this muscle works together with the psoas major muscle and is absent in 40% of the population and in some people is only on one side of the body and clinically has not much significance.

- **The Pelvic Floor:** The pelvic floor is also known as the pelvic hammock. The muscles around the pelvis floor support the pelvic organs, secured to the coccyx behind the pubis and in front of the ischial tuberosities on either side, as well as to various connective tissues structures in between

    It is very common for people to hold tension in the pelvic floor muscles along with the buttock muscles and this tension can affect the pelvic organs and cause discomfort, in such activities as bowel movements and sexual intercourse

    NOTE: some examination and treatment of these muscles can be carried out externally. When you're working the buttocks and on the perineum areas, they require an internal treatment, often through the rectum. *Internal examination and treatment on the pelvic floor muscles is an advanced, specialized technique that is beyond our scope of practice.*

The muscles of the pelvic floor are: the Coccygeus muscle and the Levator ani muscle.

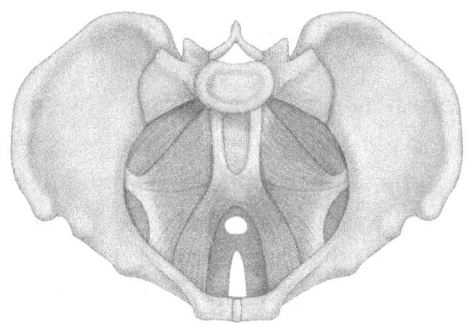

- **The Coccygeus Muscle**: the Coccygeus muscle is also known as ischiococcygeus (because it internally covers the sacrospinous ligament) and is a triangular-shaped sheet of muscle located posterior to the levator ani muscles in the pelvic floor. Together with the levator ani muscle, it forms the pelvic diaphragm.

  Its origin is in the sacrospinous ligament ischial spine, and its insertion is the coccyx and the sacrum. Its nerve is the Pudendal nerve, sacral nerve S3-S5.

  When this muscle has some trigger point pain it can travel to the coccyx, lower sacrum, and the medial aspect to the buttocks area and sometimes into the posterior hip and the leg. If the pain continues, check these muscles: the Gluteus maximus, the obturator internus, and the Quadratus Lumborum (QL).

For bonuses go to ...

Manual therapy suggestion: NOTE: first, get client's consent to work externally in this area. Lay the client in a prone position and use heat or ice to relax the area and increase the circulation. Use gentle to moderate pressure and trigger point techniques until the pain releases.

- **The Levator Ani Muscle:** its action of this muscle along with the coccygeus muscle is to resist prolapsing forces and to draw the anus upward following defecation, and to help support the pelvic viscera. NOTE: there are two parts to the levator ani: the iliac part and the pubic part. Sometimes they are also called the pubococcygeus and the iliococcygeus.

  Origin is the inner surface of the lesser pelvis and the insertion of the coccyx and center sphincter muscles and the nerve is the Pubococcygeus and Iliococcygeus.

  When there are trigger points in this muscle it can produce pain into the lower sacrum, the coccyx, and the surrounding area (buttocks). If the pain continues, check these muscles: the Gluteus maximus, the obturator internus and the Quadratus Lumborum (QL). NOTE: Manual therapy is not applied for the levator ani muscle; it cannot be externally treated.

The muscles of the posterior pelvic are: the Gluteus Maximus muscle, Gluteus Medius muscle, and Gluteus Minimus.

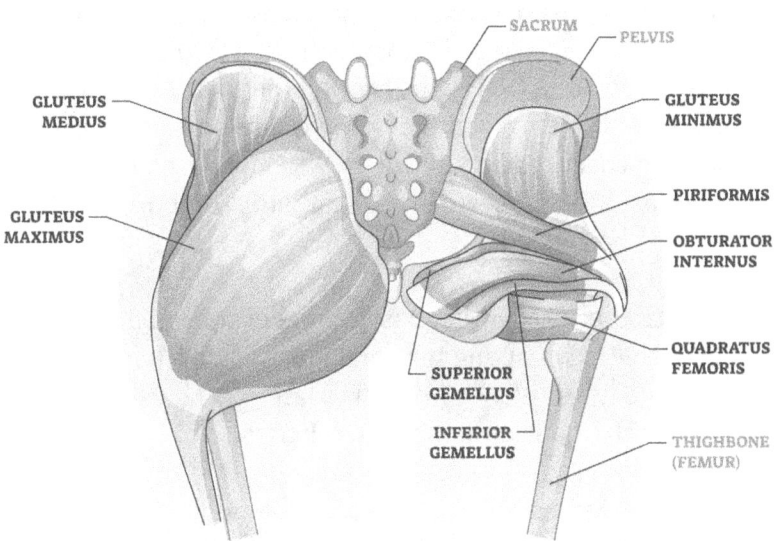

- **The Gluteus Maximus Muscle**: its action is to help with the extension of the hip during standing, to stop the pelvis from flexing forward, and to assist with the lateral rotation of the hip.

   Its origin is in the gluteus surface of ilium, the lumbar fascia, the sacrum, and the sacrotuberous ligament. Its insertion is in the gluteal tuberosity of the femur and the

Iliotibial tract. Its nerve is the Inferior gluteal nerve, L5-S2. NOTE: since gluteus maximus covers gluteus Medius and Minimus, much of the work in the buttocks applies to all three muscles, especially over the lateral aspect. The only distinction between them is the pressure applied during treatment.

When there are Trigger points in the Gluteus Maximus muscle it can cause pain from near the sacrum down to the gluteal fold. NOTE: The most common trigger point areas are the entire buttocks, the upper posterior thigh, and the coccyx region. If the pain continues, check these muscles: the Hip rotator, the Quadratus Lumborum (Q)L, and the pelvic floor.

Manual therapy suggestions: Lay the client in a prone position. Use heat and tens units to relax this (wide) area. Apply gentle stretches (medial to lateral) and use trigger point techniques until the pain releases.

- **Gluteus Medius Muscle:** its action is to abduct and to contribute with the rotation of the thigh. Also, to stabilize the pelvis while walking. Its origin is in the Gluteal surface of the Ilium, under the gluteus maximus and its insertion is in the greater trochanter of the femur. Its nerve is the Superior gluteal, L4-S1.

NOTE: The Gluteus Medius muscle together with the Gluteus Minimus is a very strong abductor of the hip, but the Minimus has far-ranging trigger points that can cause pain (in a pattern) involving the hip and the side leg down to the ankle..

When this muscle has trigger points the pain is around the buttocks area, deep into the sacrum, medial lumbar region, and into the upper posterior thigh. If the pain continues, check these muscles: Vastus Lateralis, Hamstring and Calf muscle. NOTE: The dysfunction of the Gluteus Medius is a very common cause of lower back pain.

Manual therapy suggestion: NOTE: follow the same instruction as the gluteus maximus therapy. Ask for the client's consent to be treated in this area and be mindful while draping the client (covering this area). Also, use myofascial stretch and stripping. You can have the client lie in a prone or side-lying position.

- **Gluteus Minimus Muscle:** its action is to abduct and medically (physically) rotate the thigh. Its origin is in the ilium between the anterior and inferior gluteal lines. Its insertion is to the greater trochanter of the femur and its nerve is the Superior gluteal nerve, L4-S1.

NOTE: the gluteus minimus (along with the Gluteus Medius) is a powerful abductor of the hip and it has a far ranging pain and trigger points patterns. This muscle is commonly involved in hip and leg pain. If the pain continues in this muscle, check these other muscles for trigger points: all the other gluteus muscles, the deep lateral rotators of the hip, the tensor fascia latae, the Iliotibial band, the vastus lateralis, the hamstrings and the calf muscle.

NOTE: The Gluteus Minimus muscle can mimic sciatica pain.

Massage therapy suggestions: Lay the client in a prone position and properly cover this area (draping). Use heat or ice to increase circulation and reduce tension. Use compression and friction on the attachments and trigger point techniques until the pain releases.

DEEP LATERAL ROTATORS OF THE HIP

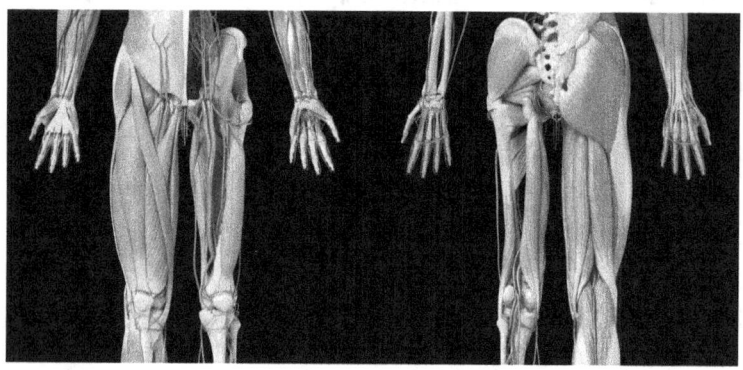

The sciatica nerve passes under, over, and through the deep lateral rotator of the hip group, especially in the Piriformis muscle area.

The muscles of the deep rotator of the hip are the Piriformis muscles, the superior Gemellus, the inferior Gemellus, the Obturator internus & the externus muscles, and the Quadratus Femoris.

- **The Piriformis Muscle:** its action is to rotate the thigh laterally and to assist with the abduction of the hip flexes and to stabilize the hip joint. Its origin is in the medial land superior to the margin of the anterior pelvic sacral foramina and the greater sciatic notch of the Ilium. Its insertion is in the lateral and inferior of the border of the greater trochanter and its nerve is the Sacral nerve, S1-S2.

NOTE: The Piriformis muscle has a profound clinical significance because it is the primary lateral rotator of the hip, as well as a stabilizer of the hip joint. One of its major dysfunction is called the Piriformis syndrome.

The Piriformis syndrome is a condition in which the piriformis muscle, located in the buttock region, spasms and causes buttock pain. The piriformis muscle also can irritate the nearby sciatic nerve and cause pain, numbness and tingling along the back of the leg and into the foot (similar to sciatic pain).

NOTE: ballet dancers have frequent problems with this muscle because of their constant demands for turnout (the rotation of the leg at the hips, which causes the feet and knees to turn outward, away from the front of the body) in ballet.

When there are trigger points in the Piriformis muscle it can cause pain that can travel over the buttock, the lateral border of the sacrum, and into the posterior thigh. By entrapment of the sciatica nerve the pain goes over the entire posterior leg, the foot, the low back, the hip, the groin, the perineum, and the rectum. If the pain continues, check these muscles for trigger points: all the gluteus muscles, the rotator of the hip, and the Quadratus Lumborum (QL).

Manual therapy suggestions: Lay the client in a prone position. Use heat or ice to reduce tension and discomfort and to improve circulation before treatment. Apply compression with stretching over the hip and petrissage strokes over the buttock area and lateral hip. Use trigger points techniques until the pain releases.

- **The Quadratus Lumborum Muscle:** The Quadratus Lumborum muscle is an overly complex and difficult muscle to treat because its anatomy attachments are inferior to the iliac crest and superior to the 12th rib and the lumbar vertebrae.

Its job is to do lateral flexion of the spine (unilateral), extension of the spine (bilateral), and to stabilize the lumbar spine. NOTE: This muscle is a troublemaker because it involves separation of movement between the upper and lower body. People that do activities like golfing, horseback riding and kayaking suffer from an intense pain in their muscles.

When there are trigger points in the Quadratus Lumborum it can cause pain in the hip, the gluteus, down to the leg, the groin, and the abdomen. If the pain continues, check these muscles: the abdominal muscles, the pelvic muscles, and the Piriformis muscle.

Manual therapy suggestion: Lay the client in a prone or side-lying position. Use heat and tens unit to induce relaxation and improve circulation to reach deep layers. First use myofascial stretch and then compression. Use trigger point techniques until the pain releases. NOTE: be careful while using friction on attachments around the 12th rib area because it can break if you apply too much force.

- **The Superior Gemellus & Inferior Gemellus Muscle:** The Superior gemellus muscle is a small muscle located deep in the posterior pelvis. Sitting underneath larger muscles of the hip and thigh, specifically to the gluteus. Its action is to rotate the thigh laterally and to stabilize the hip joint. Its origin is in the ischial spine and its margin is in the lesser sciatic notch. Its insertion is in the medial surface of the greater trochanter via the tendon of obturator internus.

The Inferior gemellus is a small, paired muscle located in the deep gluteal region of the lower extremity. It is part of a larger, tricipital (three-headed) muscle. Its origin is in the inferior gemellus muscle and the ischial tuberosity. Its insertion is in the medial surface of the greater trochanter and the tendon of the obturator internus muscle. **Note: these muscles have no clinical significance apart from the piriformis muscle.**

- **The Obturator Internus Muscle**: its action is to externally rotate the hip and to help abduct and flex the thigh. Its origin is in the ischiopubic ramus, and the obturator membrane and its insertion is in the medial aspect of the greater trochanter. Its nerve is the obturator internus nerve, L5-S1.

When there are trigger points in this muscle it can produce pain that travels mainly to the coccyx, with a less common pain pattern down the posterior thigh. If the pain continues, check these other muscles: the pelvic floor muscles, the Piriformis muscle, and the gluteus maximus muscle.

Manual therapy suggestions: Follow the same instructions as of the Piriformis muscle.

- **The Obturator Externus Muscle:** its action is to laterally rotate the thigh and to stabilize the hip joint. Its origin is in the lower half of the Obturator membrane margin and its insertion is in the trochanteric fossa of the greater trochanter. Its nerve is in the lumbosacral joint, L5-S1.

When there are trigger points in this muscle it can produce pain that travels to the medial of the lower aspect of the greater trochanter. If the pain continues, check these muscles: the Quadratus Femoris and the other deep lateral rotators of the hip, the pectineus and the adductor brevis. NOTE: the Obturator muscle may with the Quadratus Femoris cause tenderness just in the medial of the greater trochanter.

Manual therapy suggestions: Ask for client's consent to work in this area. Lay the client in a prone position. Use proper draping to cover this area. Apply compression and use trigger point techniques until the pain releases.

- **The Quadratus Femoris Muscle:** its action is to rotate the thigh laterally. Its origin is in the lateral border of the tuberosity of the Ischium and its insertion is in the Intertrochanteric crest. Its nerve is in the lumbosacral joint, L5-S1.

When this muscle produces trigger points it can cause pain similar to the Obturator externus muscle. If the pain continues, check these other muscles: the Obturator externus and the other deep lateral rotator of the hip.

Manual therapy suggestions: NOTE: you must work this muscle along with the Obturator externus (together). Ask for the client's consent to be treated in this area. Lay the client in a prone position and use proper draping. Apply compression and use trigger point techniques until the pain releases.

Muscle of the Lumbar/Lower back

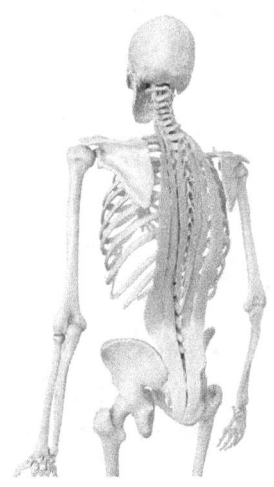

- **The Erector Spinae Group** is a term used for this group of muscles that extend and maintain the balance of the vertebral column and the rib cage. Its origin is from the sacrum, the ilium, and the processes of the lumbar vertebrae. Their insertion is in the vertebrae and the ribs. NOTE: These muscles contract very strongly when a person is coughing and they're straining during bowel movement.

    The Erector Spinae muscles are divided into three groups: **Iliocostalis, Longissimus and Spinalis.**

    Iliocostalis Group Muscles: This group represents the most lateral column of the erector Spinae. The muscles that are part of this group are: the Iliocostalis Lumborum, the Iliocostalis thoracic, and the Iliocostalis Cervicis.

- **Iliocostalis Lumborum Muscle:** its action is to extend, laterally flex, and to rotate the lumbar vertebrae. Its origin is in the sacrum and the ilium, and its insertion is in the border of the lower 6th rib. Its nerve is the posterior branch of the spinal nerve.

    When this muscle produces trigger points it can cause pain in the lumbar region into the center of the buttock. If the pain continues, check these other muscles: the erect Spinae muscles, the gluteus muscles, the Piriformis muscle, and the other hip flexors.

    Manual therapy suggestions: Lay the client in a prone position. Use heat and tens units to reduce tension and increase circulation. Apply moderate to deep pressure and do cross-fiber strokes downward. Use petrissage, deep tissue, and trigger point techniques until the pain releases.

NOTE: ask the client for feedback because working in this area is very painful.

- **Iliocostalis Thoracis Muscle:** its action is to extend, do lateral flexions, and to rotate the thoracic vertebrae. Its origin is in the medial side of the inferior borders of the lower 6th rib and its insertion is in the upper 6th rib.

NOTE: because of poor posture this muscle frequently develops painful trigger points under the scapula and the muscles of the shoulders.

When this muscle produces trigger points it can cause pain into the inside of the border of the scapula, the anterior chest, the sternum, the costal arch, the lower ipsilateral of the abdomen, and over the lumbar region. If the pain continues, check these other muscles: the trapezius, the rotator cuff muscles, the Teres major, the rhomboids, the pectoralis muscles, the Serratus posterior inferior, the Quadratus Lumborum, the abdominal obliques, and the other erect spine muscles.

Manual therapy suggestions: use the same instruction for the Iliocostalis Lumborum muscle.

- **Iliocostalis Cervicis Muscle:** its action is to extend, do lateral flexions, and to rotate the cervical vertebrae. Its origin is in the superior borders of the upper 6th rib. Its insertion is in the transverse processes of the middle cervical vertebrae. NOTE: there has not been any trigger points pain recorded for this muscle.

- **Longissimus Thoracis Muscle:** its action is to extend the vertebrae column. Its origin is in the transverse processes of the lumbar vertebrae and its insertion is in all the thoracic vertebrae and the last 10th rib.

  When this muscle produces trigger points it can cause pain over the lumbar region and into the buttock area. If the pain continues, check these other muscles: Serratus posterior inferior, Quadratus Lumborum, gluteus muscles, Piriformis, hamstrings, and the other erect Spinae muscles.

- **Spinalis Thoracis Muscle:** its action is to support and extend the vertebrae column. Its origin is in the spinous processes of the lumbar and the two lower thoracic vertebrae. Its insertion is in the spinous processes of middle and the upper thoracic vertebrae.

- **The Semispinalis Thoracis Muscle:** its action is to extend the vertebrae column. Its origin is in the transverse processes of the 5th-11th thoracic vertebrae and its insertion is in the spinous processes of the first four thoracic vertebrae and the 5th-7th cervical vertebrae. NOTE: this group of lumbar muscles are gathered together in a paraspinal bundle and it's easy to treat them together, from the posterior neck down to the sacrum (tail bone).

- **The Multifidus Muscles**: This group of muscles is located all along the vertebrae column, from the cervical region to the base of the spine. This group is one of the strongest muscles in the body and for that same reason they are subject to trigger points that can produce pain all over the lumbar region and the lower back.

  Their action is to extend, rotate, and stabilize the vertebrae column. Their origin is in the Sarum, the Iliac crest, and the vertebrae body. Their insertion is in the spinous process and their nerve is the posterior branches of the spinal nerve.

  When this muscle produces trigger points it can cause pain between the vertebrae column, the medial border of the scapula, the torso region, the upper Quadratus of the abdomen, the posterior thigh, over the sacrum, the buttock's area and the coccyx. If the pain continues, check these other muscles: the erector spinal group, the Quadratus Lumborum, the Serratus posterior inferior, the Rectus abdominis, the iliopsoas, the gluteus muscles, the hamstrings, and the abdominal obliques.

  Manual therapy suggestions: Lay the client in a prone position. Use tens units and heat or ice to reduce tension and increase circulation. Apply moderate to deep pressure and do petrissage strokes downward. Use friction on the attachments, and compression or trigger point techniques until the pain releases.

- **The Rotatores Muscles:** its action is to do bilaterally extensions of the spine, unilaterally rotation of the vertebrae and proprioception, otherwise known as kinesthesia.

Their origin is from the transverse processes of the first vertebrae and their insertion is into the root of the spine process of the next two to three vertebraes above.

NOTE: The Rotatores are the deepest layer of muscles developed in the thoracic region. Due to the abundance of muscle spindles, they probably function as organs of proprioception.

When these muscles produce pain, it goes along the midline of the spine. If the pain continues, check these other muscles: the other erector spinal group and the Multifidus muscles.

Manual therapy suggestions: Lay the client in a prone position. Use heat and a tens unit to reduce tension and increase circulation. Apply moderate to deep pressure and do cross-fiber strokes, (be very careful on cervical area). Use petrissage strokes downward, effleurage, and trigger point techniques until the pain releases. NOTE: get feedback from the client and ask if the treatment is too painful.

The muscles of the anterior thigh are: Quadriceps Femoris, Vastus Anterior, Vastus Lateralis, Vastus Intermedius, Rectus Femoris.

This group of muscles is on the anterior thigh across the hip and the knee joint. Their job is to extend the knee, flex the hips at the Rectus Femoris muscle.

When there are trigger points in the Vastus Medius muscle it can cause pain to the anterior thigh and the knee. Trigger points in the Vastus Lateralis muscle can cause pain to the lateral thigh and L- knee. If the pain continues, check these other muscles: the hip adductors, the tensor fasciae latae (TFL) and the Iliotibial band (ITB), and the Obturator internus muscle.

Manual therapy suggestions: Lay the client in a supine position. Use heat and tens unit to prepare this large group of muscles for treatment. Apply compression and cross-fiber friction around the patella and the tendons around the knee. Use friction in attachments, stripping, petrissage and trigger point techniques until the pain releases. NOTE: If a client had knee surgery you need doctor consent to do a massage treatment.

The other anterior thigh muscle is the Sartorius. NOTE: A great high light information is when this muscle is tight the piriformis muscle stretches. If there are trigger points in this muscle it can cause pain in the Quadriceps, and the hip adductors.

Manual therapy suggestions: use the same techniques for the Quadricep group and remember to apply strokes upward.

- **The Muscle of the Posterior Thigh:** it is also called Hamstrings and they originate at the Semitendinosus and attaches from the ischial tuberosity to the medial tibia, Bicep Femoris, lateral to the head of the fibula, and the

Semimembranosus medial condyle of the tibia. Their job is to extend the hip, flex the knee and to rotate the knee in medially (toward the middle or center) when it's flexed.

When there are trigger points in the muscle of the posterior thigh it can cause pain at the back of the leg, from buttocks to the mid-calf. If the pain continues, check these other muscles: The quadratus lumborum (QL), the Piriformis muscle, the Gluteal group, and the hip adductors.

Manual therapy suggestions: NOTE: be very cautious not to apply pressure into the popliteal space behind the knee. Lay the client in a prone position. Use heat and tens units to prepare this large area. Apply compression, do cross friction on the attachments and use strokes upward. Use trigger point techniques until the pain releases. Do gentle stretches after the treatment.

- **The Lateral Thigh Muscles:** are the Tensor Fasciae Latae (TFL) and the Iliotibial Band (IT). These muscles' fibers are fibrous, and they extend from the crest of the Ilium to the lateral condyle of the tibia. Together they help flex, abduct, and medially rotate the hip.

The IT Band is controlled by the TFL and the Gluteus Maximus. When there are trigger points in these muscles it can cause pain that radiates to the lateral aspect of the thigh. If the pain continues, check the Vastus Lateralis muscle.

Manual therapy suggestions: Lay the client in a supine position. Use heat and a tens unit on the quadriceps. Apply compression, stripping, petrissage, and trigger point technique until the pain releases.

- **The Muscle of the Medial Thigh (Hip Adductor):** This nickname almost gives away its function and it also collaborates with flexion, extension, rotation, and stability of the hips while standing, walking, or climbing. The muscle of the medial thigh (Hip Adductor) attaches to the pubis and into the ischial tuberosity, the Adductor Magnus, the Adductor Longus, the Adductor Brevis, the Pectineus and the Gracilis.

    When there are trigger points in the muscle of the medial thigh (Hip Adductor) it can cause pain to the medial aspect of the thigh.

    Manual therapy suggestions: Lay the client in a supine position or the side lowering the leg straight. Apply compression, do friction by the knee and use trigger point techniques until the pain releases.

- **Connective Tissues of the Legs and Feet:** Ligaments are strong connective tissues connecting bones to other bones, forming joints. The leg muscles are tough and elastic tissues that hold the bones of the feet.

    The foot's job is to do an external and internal rotation, inversion, and eversion (supination and pronation) movements like running. These movements are precisely what the muscles of the legs and feet coordinate.

For bonuses go to ...

When all these movements are chronic, they create dysfunctions and require immediate attention.

Do not be fooled; these structures are more complex because they combine the legs, the ankles, and their feet. Their job is weight bearing forward of the ankle and for that main reason the ankles are very vulnerable when there is a bad alignment or a bad posture. NOTE: The calf muscle is constantly working (moving), creating trigger points and dysfunctions that travel to the rest of the body.

Manual therapy suggestions: NOTE: Keep in mind the foot positions when you are doing your massage treatment. Remember that the ankle joint does not like to move to lateral or medial position.

NOTE: The leg and the ankle are anatomical complex, and we must pay attention to every connective tissue, like the Crural Fascia, which attaches from the knee, the medial collateral ligament, the patellar ligament, the fascia lata, the extensor retinaculum superior and inferior. The proper massage treatment is to apply deep strokes and friction to free the structures of the leg.

- **Flexor Retinaculum:** is a wide band crossing the medial malleolus to the medial and upper board of the calcaneus, and the plantar surface as far as the navicular bone. It holds in place the tendons of the tibialis posterior, the flexor digitorum longus, and the flexor hallucis longus.

The Inferior Extensor Retinaculum is a Y shape ligament, and its job is to restrain the extensor tendons of the foot.

The Superior Extensor Retinaculum is a ligament that binds the extensor tendons proximal to the ankle joint. It has two fibrous bands that retain the tendons of the peroneus longus and the brevis.

Manual therapy suggestions: Lay the client in a supine position. Use heat to make this area more responsive to pressure and friction. Use gentle stretches after treatment.

- **Plantar Fascia (Plantar Aponeurosis)**: it's a very thick fascia in the plantar muscle and attaches the flexor muscles to the toes. The Plantar Fascia (Plantar Aponeurosis) Trigger points pain radiates to the toes.

  Manual therapy suggestion: Lay the client in a prone position. NOTE: make sure to support the ankle with a pillow or bolster. Use heat on calf muscles and apply friction, petrissage, and thumb compression with upward strokes. Use gentle stretches after treatment.

- **Tibialis Anterior:** The tibialis anterior muscle is a muscle in humans that originates along the upper two-thirds of the lateral (outside) surface of the tibia and inserts into the medial cuneiform and the first metatarsal bones of the foot. It acts to dorsiflex and invert the foot. This muscle is mostly located near the shin.

  When there are trigger points in the tibialis anterior muscle it can cause pain in the anterior aspect of the ankle toward the big toe. If the pain continues, check these other muscles: the Extensor Hallucis Longus.

Manual therapy suggestions: NOTE: this area is very painful. So, ask the client for feedback, as much as you can. Lay the client in a supine position. Use heat from the knee down to the ankle to make the muscles more subjected to treatment and to release tension. Stabilize the foot while working on this muscle and use compression, friction upward, effleurage and trigger point techniques until the pain releases.

- **Extensor Digitorum Longus:** Extensor Digitorum Longus is posterior to the tibialis anterior covering the fibula and ends at the second to the fifth toes, remember these muscles have small tendons as attachments.

  When there are trigger points in the Extensor Digitorum Longus muscle it can cause pain at the top of the foot and into the second, third, and fourth digits (toes). If the pain continues, check these other muscles: the Extensor Digitorum brevis.

  Manual therapy suggestions: use the same instructions as the Tibialis Anterior muscle.

- **Extensor Hallucis Longus:** Extensor hallucis longus muscle is a thin muscle that extends from the middle third of the fibula to the distal phalanx of the big toe (hallux). The muscle belongs to the anterior compartment of the leg together with three other muscles: extensor digitorum longus, tibialis anterior and fibularis tertius muscles.

  The extensor hallucis longus specifically extends the hallux, dorsiflexes the foot at the ankle, and inverts the foot. The extensor hallucis longus muscle is susceptible to several pathologies, including nerve injury resulting in foot drop, tendonitis, tendon rupture, and anterior compartment syndrome.

Peroneus Longus, Brevis & Tertius Muscle Group:

In human anatomy, the fibularis longus (also known as peroneus longus) is a superficial muscle in the lateral compartment of the leg. It acts to tilt the sole of the foot away from the midline of the body (eversion) and to extend the foot downward away from the body (plantar flexion) at the ankle. The peroneus brevis muscle is the shorter of the two muscles that make up the lateral compartment of the leg, with the peroneus longus being the longer muscle. The function of the peroneus brevis muscle is to evert the foot and plantarflex the ankle.

The Peroneus Tertius muscle, also called Fibularis Tertius, is one of the 3 peroneal muscles (peroneus longus, Peroneus Brevis). [1] It is the most superficial muscle in the anterior compartment of the leg.

Manual therapy suggestions: use the same instructions as the Tibialis Anterior muscle.

The posterior muscles of the leg are:

- **The Popliteus Muscles:** is located behind the lateral of the knee and the tibia, by the soleal line. NOTE: be very careful around this area because the tibial nerves and the popliteal artery are nearby.

When there are trigger points in the Popliteus muscles it can cause pain behind the knee. If the pain continues, check the Gastrocnemius muscle.

Manual therapy suggestions: Lay the client in a prone or sideways position (lying on the unaffected leg). Apply compression, friction on attachments, effleurage, and trigger point techniques until the pain releases. Use gentle stretches after treatment.

- **The Gastrocnemius Muscles:** it crosses the knee, and the ankle joint by the Achilles tendon. Its job is to plantar flexion the foot. NOTE: Plantar flexion is the movement that allows you to press the gas pedal of your car.

When there are trigger points in the Gastrocnemius muscles it can cause pain to the ankle down to the arch of the foot. If the pain continues, check the Piriformis muscle.

- **The Soleus Muscles:** is the number one muscle related to pain in the heel. It originates under the gastrocnemius muscle by the shaft of the fibula, soleal line, the medial margin of the tibia, and the calcaneus. Its action is to plantar flexion of the foot.

When there are trigger points in the Soleus muscles it can cause pain over the Achilles tendon to the plantar surface of the heel. If the pain continues, check the Quadratus plantae muscle.

Manual therapy suggestions: Lay the client in a prone position. Use heat and tens unit by the feet. Apply compression and friction on the Achilles tendon and the attachments. Use deep tissue on the whole posterior leg and trigger point techniques until the pain releases. Use gentle stretches after the treatment.

- **The Plantaris Muscle:** NOTE: this is a very tricky muscle to work on. Be aware of its small sizes and the long tendon passing next to the Achilles tendon, which is attached to the deep fascia of the ankle

  Its action is to assist the plantar flexion of the foot. When there are trigger points in the Plantaris muscles it can cause pain behind the knee and the upper calf. If the pain continues, check these other muscles: the Soleus and the Piriformis.

- **The Tibialis Posterior Muscle:** this muscle is one of the deep layers of the posterior leg. Its origin is between the tibia, the fibula, and the interosseous membrane, which is attached to the navicular, the three cuneiform cuboids, and the second, third and fourth toes. Its action is to plantar flex and the inversion of the foot. If there are trigger points for pain in these muscles, also check the muscles of the posterior leg.

  Manual therapy suggestions: use the same instructions as the Tibialis Anterior muscle.

- **Flexor Digitorum Longus:** The other deep layer is the Flexor Digitorum Longus, which flexes the second to the fifth toes

When there are trigger points in the Flexor Digitorum Longus it can cause pain to the medial calf, the central plantar surface, the Hallucis Longus muscle that flexes the big toe, the ball of the foot and the great toe. If the pain continues, check all the posterior leg muscles. Manual therapy suggestions: use the same instructions as the Tibialis Anterior muscle.

- **The Muscles of the Feet**: small in size but extraordinarily strong. Its origin starts at the Quadratus Plantae muscle, found deep and close to the calcaneus (heel). It also attaches on the tendons of the flexor muscles and assists with the flexion of the foot. When there are trigger points in the muscles of the feet it can cause pain to the plantar aspect of the heel. If the pain continues, check the Soleus muscle.

- **The Flexor Digiti Minimi Brevis:** The flexor digiti minimi brevis (foot) is a muscle that is located on the outer edge of the foot bones. It begins at the fifth metatarsal (the bone behind the bones of the pinky toe) and sheath of the peroneus longus muscle, located in the sole of the foot. Its action is to flex the little toe.

- **The Flexor Digitorum Brevis:** The flexor digitorum brevis is a muscle which lies in the middle of the sole of the foot, immediately above the central part of the plantar aponeurosis, with which it is firmly united. Its deep surface is separated from the lateral plantar vessels and nerves by a thin layer of fascia.

NOTE: this muscle is right at the center of the plantar fascia of the foot, flexes the fourth toes.

When there are trigger points in the Flexor Digitorum Brevis it can cause pain to the middle of the sole of the foot and into the toes.

- **The Flexor Hallucis Brevis:** Flexor hallucis brevis (FHB) is one of the muscles in the third layer (of four layers) of plantar muscles. It is located adjacent to the plantar surface of the 1st metatarsal and contains 2 sesamoid bones. NOTE: it is in an angle position at the cuboid bone and attaches to the base of the big toe.

When there are trigger points in the Flexor Hallucis Brevis it can cause pain in the ball of the foot into the big toe, and into both sides of the foot.

- **The Extensor Digitorum Brevis:** Extensor digitorum brevis is a thin muscle found on the dorsum of the foot. This region contains the dorsal compartment of the foot, which houses extensor digitorum brevis and extensor hallucis brevis. These muscles are covered by the deep dorsal fascia of the foot.

NOTE: it is on top of the foot and from the calcaneus it's attached by four tendons to the base of the phalanx (toes) next to the big toe.

When there are trigger points in the Extensor Digitorum Brevis it can cause pain into the top of the foot and the outside of the ankle.

- **The Abductor Hallucis:** its origin is from the inside area of the calcaneus to the big toe. Trigger points in this muscle can cause pain at the arch of the foot and the pain can spillover to the Gastrocnemius muscle. NOTE: The Adductor Hallucis has two heads: the oblique and the transverse. They cover the metatarsophalangeal joints to the lateral side of the great toe.

- **The Abductor Digiti Minimi:** This muscle originates from the lateral heel to the case of the pinky toe. Trigger points in this muscle can cause pain in the outer edge of the foot.

- **Lumbrical Muscles and the Interosseous Muscles:** Other muscles of the foot are the Lumbrical muscles, and the Interosseous muscles located in between the base of the toes. When there are trigger points in these muscles it can cause pain in the dorsal and the plantar of the foot. Manual therapy suggestions for these groups of muscles is to lay the client in a supine position. Apply moderate pressure and use friction and effleurage to induce relaxation.

PROGRESS

Measuring progress, effectiveness, and outcomes helps determine when treatment is done and when a client has achieved what they wanted from the massage therapy and the treatment can end.

How to Track Client Progress

- Progress reports. Structured progress reports are a simple and effective means of helping clients evaluate progress and focus on their goals.
- Before and after photos. Sometimes a simple visual reminder can speak volumes.
- Workout or nutrition records.
- Communication.

Why do you think it's important to measure client progress?

It is essential to measure a client's progress because when people are in pain all they know is that the pain is still present, and they lose perspective of their own progress. In every visit, I write in their chart notes about their pain level when they perform their Activities of Daily Living (ADLs). This information helps me determine if they are making better choices to contribute to their health and if the massage treatment is helping them improve.

How has measuring client progress can help you grow your practice?

Clients see how effective massage therapy is in their healing and in their quality of life. Massage offers relief and measuring that progress is the key to maintaining hope that more permanent relief is possible.

What tools do you use for measuring client progress?

The easiest tool to use is a 0-10 scale to rate pain and function. This can be assessed verbally and often and can be graphed to demonstrate progress over time. In addition, there are many scales that provide descriptions of daily activities, asking the user to check a phrase that most accurately describes their ability to perform the activity. These include the Functional Rating Index, the Oswestry or Vernon-Mior Pain and Disability Index to name a few.

What advice do you have for a massage therapist who is interested in getting better at tracking client progress?

Start with one patient this week that has pain and some loss of normal function and ask them to rate their pain and function on a scale of 0 (no pain) and 10 (worst pain imaginable). Next, pick one more person and do the same thing. Keep it up each time the person returns, ask them to rate their pain and function, and begin comparing the numbers to previous sessions. If you add one person per week, you gradually get better at tracking and eventually you will be tracking progress for everyone.

Notes

PHASE 2

Chapter 8

Breaking the Pattern of Dysfunction & Imbalance

Massage Routine or Evolving Treatment

If your client does not have any relief after three treatments go back and review your notes and study the case again; get involved. Our goal is to get them out of pain and dysfunction so do not get stuck doing the same treatment, especially if you do not see results or progress. Re-evaluate the client's condition, change the treatment plan if it is necessary and evolve into a more appropriate modality. Also make sure the client is following your recommendations because it can hinder their progress if they are not. Keep in mind that a massage alone may not be enough. For example, the client could need more physical activity or more rest. The goal is to treat the client to get better and just in need of maintenance treatment, which is usually once a month treatment for three to four months.

Adaptation

We are going to encounter surprises after a few treatments. The body will shift, and it will try to adjust to the newest patterns. So do not get discouraged if it's taking longer than expected to see results or progress. In some cases, this is very normal, especially after the client had surgery, because the body as whole is healing. After an assessment, see if a different modalities and sequence of treatment is necessary. Make sure to always adapt your treatments in search of the best solution to heal your clients!

Management of Complex Conditions

Massage can reduce pain and anxiety for people with chronic illnesses, such as cancer, and reduce the physiological burden of stress. It can help treat conditions including stress-related tension, cancer-related fatigue, sleep disorders, high blood pressure, diabetes, low back pain and depression, just to name a few.

Serious and persistent chronic conditions are **multidimensional, interdependent, complex, and ongoing**. Chronic conditions are characterized by persistent and recurring health consequences lasting for three months or more.

Enhance Your Skills

Here are a couple suggestions on how you can enhance your skills as a massage therapy professional:

- **Expand Your Knowledge:** Are there any new techniques you are not aware of that could benefit your clients? I recommend you to learn orthopedic massage and kinesiology therapy because they are essential modalities.
- **Provide a Relaxing Workspace:** Outside noises and disturbances should be quelled. Essential oils are great for soothing the client's senses along with other massage oils. The warmth of stone, bamboo and warm towels also relax the client. There are many things that are simple and inexpensive to add to the relaxed atmosphere of a massage.
- **Practice Good Hygiene:** A massage therapist should wash their hands for about 20-30 seconds before and after each massage. Washing before and after each massage ensures that their hands are clean for each massage, and it prevents the spread of germs.
- **Focus on Your Clients:** Being compassionate, spending appropriate time with patients, demonstrating active listening, and helping to advise and resolve the patient's problems will all contribute to building a trusting, respectful relationship.
- **Provide Excellent Customer Service:** A massage therapist with excellent customer service skills will not just make an impression on their clients–they will also allow their clients to make an impression on them. Learn a client's health history and the concerns that brought them in, but also pay attention to the client's stories. I invite you to expand

your knowledge and to keep up with your continual education. The more knowledgeable you are, the more powerful and successful you become!

Analysis and Interpretation

While gathering information from the client, the massage therapist must interpret the data provided to determine the best and safest treatment strategy to meet the client's needs.

I am sharing my knowledge and experiences and offering this book as guidance for every therapist who reads it and applies it. Now, if you do not know something we have avenues to find information; studies and research have been done for us. I encourage you to get a mentor you can shadow in different situations, as it's easier that way for you to learn new skills. Some people learn visually, or by dictation; find your way.

Outcomes, Methods & Variations

There is much massage research and studies that prove the effectiveness of massage therapists in pain management. More than 500 million people are affected by pain and headaches and back pain are the most listed. Clearly, there are so many people in need of a massage treatment and therefore, our job as massage therapists can be the solution for treating these conditions. This is exactly why we learn, study, and prepare ourselves with the necessary training and certification to acquire the skills to help improve our modalities and techniques as massage therapists and practitioners.

Notes

Chapter 9

Listen, Observe & Feel

Subjective and Objective Symptoms

- **Subjective**: information about the client's own description of their chief complaint.
- **Objective**: observable and measurable information about the client's current symptoms gathered by the massage therapist and other professionals.

Assessment: identifying the client's condition and analysis of their progress. People tend to change their mind about their personal interpretation in regard to their pain or what is going on with them in general. Share your professional opinion and keep records of factual data.

Measurement of Progress

In our profession it is very difficult to measure progress apart from getting inside from our client's opinion and perspective. There are basic tools we can use like the **Goniometer** to measure the angles of the joints to determine the Range of Motion (ROM). To measure the alignment of the body, using an **Inclinometer** works like a spirit level, the carpenter tool used to indicate how parallel (level) or perpendicular (plumb) a surface is relative to the earth. The other one is the PALM (**Palpation meter**) before and after treatment; keep records of your progress for future references. The medical community is very constrained on claiming any results without scientific research or studies. It is interesting to know that new scientific research is available today regarding the benefits of a massage. I invite you to read some of these amazing materials and research published by the Massage Therapy Foundation and the International Journal of Therapeutic Massage & Bodywork (IJTMB).

Habits Contributing to the Current Situation

Our awareness of the client's complaints, present problems, health history, athletic history, personal and social history, and of course occupational history will guide us to better choices of treatment and to choose areas for more scrutiny. We need to be an initiative-taker, like investigators to find the source of our clients' pain, discomfort, and suffering.

Treatment Plan or Referral Out

If the client is not getting better with the treatments, or you are stuck and have used all the techniques and different modalities you know and nothing has worked, then you must consider referring your client to his/her healthcare physician for an extensive evaluation to find out why he/she is not getting better and what further treatment and medical attention he/she might need. Be honest and sincere with yourself if their symptoms and conditions are beyond your scope of practice. Do not be discouraged! On the contrary, take it as gaining wisdom, knowledge, and experience for facing these difficult cases.

On Call or Not

Outcall massage service is a business which provides massage at a location designated by the client or the massage practitioner or therapist, other than at a massage establishment.

You will need to determine if you are willing to provide services after business hours or be on call for a selective client(s).

Client Packages

I use package deals mainly for clients I know will need multiple treatment sessions within several weeks. This can be used for brand new clients after an assessment visit or an established client that only needs maintenance treatments.

Here is where you can decide to keep treating the clients and book them in your schedule ahead of time and offer a special discount as an appreciation.

For bonuses go to www.AwildaPelaezLMT.com

Notes

Chapter 10

You Are Your Business

Results Get You Referrals!

Write Your Business Plan

Starting a business takes research, intelligence, self-confidence, diligence, responsibility, and guts to face your fears. Your company should cover the history and nature of your business. A business plan is an objective statement that spells out exactly what you would like to accomplish in the near term and over the long term.

A well-written plan should include details about your business goals, services, and finances. Your company should be registered and should also have a defined business structure such as a sole proprietorship, partnership, or corporation. Make sure to consult a CPA for assistance in making your decisions.

The US Small Business Administration or the Small Business Development centers provide free business consulting and help with business plan development and can also be a resource for you.

Marketing Plan

Do the basics, make business cards, do market research in your area and discover what sets you apart from the competition. Analyze your competitors, and what they do well, then point out what you can do better.

You can address how you plan to persuade customers to pay for your services, and how you will develop customer loyalty that will lead to repeat business, by joining a networking group or a chamber of commerce in your area, which will help you meet new potential clients.

Pick a Location

If you are a startup, you may have to work for somebody else in the beginning, and it can be a blessing in disguise because you will be in an established business already. On the other hand, if you have the finances to start on your own, maybe renting a room in a chiropractic office or another massage therapy is a good choice because you can be referred business directly from these medical providers. Another great location could be a Health club or gyms because the clientele are people that invest in their health.

Insurance

A business needs insurance because it helps cover the cost associated with property damage and liability claims. There are different types of business insurance, including property damage insurance, legal liability insurance and employment practice liability insurance.

Property insurance provides financial reimbursement to the owner or renter of a structure and its contents in case there is damage or theft, and to a person other than the owner or renter if that person is injured on the property.

Liability insurance helps cover medical and legal fees if you are held legally responsible for someone else's injury or damage to someone else's property.

Employment practice liability insurance (EPLI) includes coverage for defense cost and damages relates to various employment-related claims including allegations of wrongful termination, discrimination, workplace harassment and retaliation.

The American Massage Therapy Association (AMTA) has some insurance policies available for massage therapists.

Get Your Business Tax ID and Register Your business

Your employer identification number (EIN) is an important step to start and grow your business, like opening a business bank account and paying taxes. Even if you can use your social security number for your business, the states require you to get a tax ID as well.

Keep your business running smoothly by staying legally compliant. The licenses and permits you need for your business will vary by industry, state, location, and other factors.

Open a Business Account and a Line of Credit

A small business account can help you handle legal, taxes and day to day transactions. It's easy to set one up if you have the right registrations and paperwork ready. Funding your business will help you figure out how much money you will need to start your business; fortunately, there are more ways than ever to find capital you need.

Build a Website and Blog

A business website generally serves as a space to provide general information about your company or a direct platform for e-commerce. Keep it simple but with good substance and elements. For example: A clear purpose, a simple web address, strong & professional branding, easy to find contact information, strong call to action and compelling content.

Set Schedule for Self-Care

Self-care is the practice of taking an active role in protecting one's own well-being and happiness, in particular during periods of stress. Remember to preserve and improve your own health. Invest in activities that promote good behaviors and active management of illness when it occurs. Engage in some form of self-care daily with food choice, exercise, sleep, and dental care.

There are 7 pillars of Self-Care:

* The Mental pillar of self-care is about cultivating a healthy mindset through mindfulness and curiosity.
- The Emotional pillar of self-care involves taking care of your heart with healthy coping strategies.
- The Physical pillar of self-care encompasses any processes or activities that affect your physical well-being, including diet choices, exercise, and sleep patterns.
- The Environmental pillar of self-care involves taking care of the spaces and places around you.
- The Spiritual pillar of self-care involves activities or practices that give a sense of meaning to your life.
- The Recreational pillar of self-care involves making time for hobbies, fun activities, and new experiences.
- The Social pillar of self-care involves building relationships with regular connection and healthy boundaries.

Body Language

Keep in mind that when a client or patient comes in they may be in distress and extremely uncomfortable. How you react to them can create either a negative or positive impression, and your body language cannot fake your attitude.

Be Polite and Courteous

Being polite is showing behavior that is respectful toward others, especially in the healthcare setting. Showing your good bedside manners show who you really are as a human being. Make sure that you are courteous at every interaction.

Set the Tone and Show Interest

Carry yourself with authority, without arrogance or a sense of importance, when you are dealing with clients in or outside your practice. You do not want to be perceived as a rude or grumpy person, but approachable, genuine and friendly!

Be Grateful and Respectful

Always be considerate of others and treat everyone with respect and dignity. Also be thankful for the opportunity of helping your clients in their health journey. Every client is different so every experience will be different. Massage therapist is a very satisfying career when we do it from the heart!

Punctuality

Punctuality is a major key to success because you are ready to take and respect your business and clients by being on time.

Appreciation

Recognize the full value of each person crossing your door and each opportunity they represent, because one client has the potential to connect you to a thousand people and launch your business by referring you to others, which is priceless.

Notes

About the Author

Awilda Pelaez was born in the Dominican Republic and moved to Long Island, New York in 1994. She has been the proud owner of a remarkably successful private practice for over twelve years.

Here is a little bit of her story: When she was about five years old, Awilda suffered a tragic bicycle accident, breaking her left fibula and tibia bones. She was truly blessed to be aided and treated by a neighbor who happened to be a retired nurse, named Altagracia, aka Tata, who believed in the healing power of a medical massage.

It took about 6 months for Awilda to be completely healed. This experience was the seed of inspiration for her and, even though she was a child, she was impacted by Tata's care, knowledge, skills, and compassion. It has been 40 years since that date and Awilda is still able to use her legs without any pain.

This is the reason why Awilda became a medical massage practitioner, so she can help others the same way she was helped.

The author is available to participate in conferences, seminars, and keynote presentations. For more information about her rates and availability, please contact Awilda directly at http://learnsofttissuemanipulationskillsbook.com/

www.ingramcontent.com/pod-product-compliance
Lightning Source LLC
Chambersburg PA
CBHW071402210526
45465CB00001B/209